Wired for Intimacy. How pornography hijacks the male brain. By William M. Struthers.

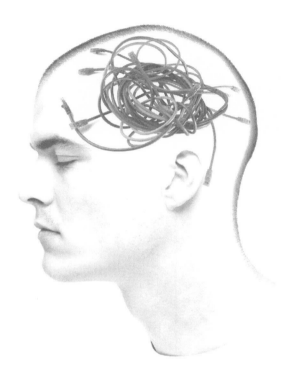

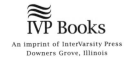

IVP Books

An imprint of InterVarsity Press
Downers Grove, Illinois

InterVarsity Press
P.O. Box 1400, Downers Grove, IL 60515-1426
World Wide Web: www.ivpress.com
E-mail: email@ivpress.com

InterVarsity Press® is the book-publishing division of InterVarsity Christian Fellowship/USA®, a movement of students and faculty active on campus at hundreds of universities, colleges and schools of nursing in the United States of America, and a member movement of the International Fellowship of Evangelical Students. For information about local and regional activities, write Public Relations Dept., InterVarsity Christian Fellowship/USA, 6400 Schroeder Rd., P.O. Box 7895, Madison, WI 53707-7895, or visit the IVCF website at <www.intervarsity.org>.

While all stories in this book are true, some names and identifying details have been changed to protect the privacy of those involved.

Figure 4.2 on p. 91 is from David G. Myers, Psychology, ninth edition (figure 2.33). New York: Worth Publishers. ©2010 by Worth Publishers. Used by permission.

Design: Cindy Kiple
Images: tangled ethernet cables: Influx Productions/Getty Images
*   profile of man's head: PhotoAlto/Alix Minde/Getty Images*

ISBN 978-0-8308-3700-7

Printed in the United States of America ∞

Library of Congress Cataloging-in-Publication Data

Struthers, William M., 1970-
  Wired for intimacy: how pornography hijacks the male brain/
  William Struthers.
     p. cm.
  Includes bibliographical references.
  ISBN 978-0-8308-3700-7 (pbk.: alk. paper)
  1. Pornography—Religious aspects—Christianity 2. Sex
  addiction—Religious aspects—Christianity. 3. Men—Psychology. 4.
  Sex differences (Psychology) 5. Brain—Sex differences. I. Title.
  BV4597.6.S77 2009
  241'.667—dc22

                                           2009032133

P 25 24 23 22 21 20 19 18 17 16 15 14 13 12

Y 30 29 28 27 26 25 24 23 22 21 20 19 18 17 16

For every man who longs to be known as holy and good.

Contents

Acknowledgments

THERE ARE MANY INDIVIDUALS whom I would like to thank for their help and encouragement in the writing of this book. First my wife, Donna, who during a rush hour trip to her parents with the kids asleep in the van challenged me to offer a course on men and addictions at Wheaton College. Second, those at InterVarsity Press and InterVarsity Christian Fellowship who have helped me along the way: my editor, Al Hsu, who provided me with keen insight and feedback, and Roger Anderson, who arranged for the pornography workshop and speaking opportunities to share what men needed to hear. And finally my friends, students and colleagues who took time to help me proof chapters and let me bounce ideas off of them. You know who you are, and I am humbled by your encouragement.

Introduction

WHAT IS IT ABOUT PORNOGRAPHY that makes it so appealing to so many men? Why does a naked female body or a movie of a woman having sex seem to hijack a man's brain, hypnotizing him and rendering him incapable of making good decisions? Why might a man who is married to a lovely wife risk that relationship for a ten-second video clip of a couple having sex? What is it about being male that makes it so difficult for men to look away?

While pornography ravages and destroys the lives of both men and women, this book and the research within focuses almost exclusively on pornography's impact on men. It is true that women are increasingly becoming consumers of pornography, but there is little doubt that it is primarily men who are hooked on it. And the reasons that women view pornography are very different than the reasons men do. Men seem to be wired in such a way that pornography hijacks the proper functioning of their brains and has a long-lasting effect on their thoughts and lives.

As a biopsychologist and a person of faith, I am in a unique position to engage many of the questions posed above. It is hard to be a Christian in the United States and not be sensitive to the pervasive influence of pornography and the warped views of sexuality that saturate our culture. Pornography and the hypersexuality found in the media are almost impossible to avoid.

As I have looked more carefully at some of my Christian beliefs about sexuality and felt convicted to respond to the pornification of our culture, I have had an unexpected opportunity to integrate my faith with my academic discipline. As I have studied how the brain develops, how hormones and culture affect it and how addictions and compulsions develop, it has become increasingly apparent to me why many men struggle so much. In this book I share this material, and I hope it can be a part of the healing process that so many long for.

Like many adolescent boys growing up in the 1980s, I had occasional opportunities to view lingerie catalogs in the mail and softcore pornography magazines stashed away by friends and relatives. These were my first exposures to the naked female form, eliciting what I now know to be sexual interest. As I grew older, frontal nudity and erotic sexual scenes in movies became readily viewable on cable television channels such as HBO and Playboy. Home videotapes made access to all types of pornography easier than ever before.

While I can't recall feeling a compelling attraction toward pornography, I won't deny that I found it hypnotizing when I stumbled upon it. But I was struck by the hold that it had over several of my teenage friends and their desire to expose me to it. Perhaps I was just late in my sexual awakening, but as I entered my twenties, my exposure to porn shifted into high gear. Legally an adult and living with other men who were enjoying the freedoms of college life, I was exposed to additional forms of pornography. I became increasingly aware of how many men subscribed to *Playboy* and regularly rented adult videos. I began to notice how many of my friends and acquaintances—men who by all other accounts would have made fine boyfriends and husbands—sacrificed relationships with real women for the allure of an image of a woman on the magazine page or videotape of a couple having sex. I admit that I was not a saint and did not avert my eyes from every temptation. I believe that it is only by the grace of God that I was mostly spared from the seductive draw of the pornographic page and screen.

I can think of many ways I have benefited from computer technologies and the vast knowledge available on the Internet. But I also delete dozens of e-mails each day that solicit pornographic material, sexual enhancement products or opportunities for sexual encounters. My workplace has an Internet filter, but sexually explicit material is easy to access if you are determined. I put on self-imposed blinders as I wade through tantalizing advertisements with Victoria's Secret models in the margins of my weather forecast. My Internet service provider's homepage is littered with dating services ("Hot Single Girls in Your Neighborhood Looking for Love!") and my sports websites have galleries of scantily clad cheerleaders. If I watch a soccer match on television with my children, I have to be vigilant to change the channel when commercials for Viagra are aired. In a world that has been hypersexualized, it is hard to get through the day without being battered and numbed by the intrusions of pornography.

Many people have asked me if I have ever looked at pornography. I'm not sure if the question is geared to label me a hypocrite or to appeal to an "everybody does it" mentality. When I tell them that I find many things on television or on newsstands pornographic, they frown. Apparently this makes me a prude, which is worse than being a hypocrite. Yes, I have viewed pornography because *it is everywhere.* You cannot get away from it; if you don't view it intentionally, you will unintentionally. The result is that repeated exposure to pornography and the objectification of the female body changes the way our brains see each other. Repeated exposure to any stimulus results in neurological circuit making. That is how we learn. But what does pornography teach and how does it change those who regularly consume it?

My journey in asking this question began several years ago when, as a faculty member at a Christian college, two significant things happened. First, I knew three men in different stages of life and from varied backgrounds who had problems with pornography and engaged in sexually inappropriate behaviors. These men had allowed pornography to warp their idea of sexuality, impacting them and their families negatively. Watching these men deal with the consequences of their problems was exceptionally painful. In one situation, I felt that I had unknowingly contributed to the breakdown of one man's marriage by encouraging him to discover the wonders of the Internet for quick and easy stock trading. Instead he discovered it as a gateway to free pornography and depravity.

A second factor was an upper-division psychology class I taught called Men and Addictions. In part of this course, I spent a significant amount of time exploring findings about men's struggles with pornography and compulsive sexual behaviors. We evaluated whether or not a person could become addicted to porn and if it should be classified as a clinical problem. This component to the course turned out to be an invitation for hordes of college-aged men to visit me during my office hours. There they confided that they felt trapped by their inability to stop consuming pornography. The weight of the guilt they carried was heartbreaking.

I began the process of seeking out therapeutic options for these men and came across statistics about the adult entertainment industry. I was flabbergasted at the economics and demographics of it all. I met regularly with these young men and referred them to counselors when appropriate. It became apparent that many of them were dealing with significant emotional and spiritual wounds that had resulted from their experience with pornography. This book is a result of the great need for healing that I saw in these men as a result of pornography consumption.

My personal agenda will be clearly evident to anyone who reads this book. It stems from my Christian faith and my desire that each person fully understand how we all are unique and appreciate how much we share in common as human beings created in the image of God. My faith requires that every human life be viewed as sacred and the dignity of every individual be respected and honored. When we better understand the devastating spiritual, psychological, social and biological reality of how pornography violates our unique position in God's creation, we will be better able to minister to those who have been wounded by it.

Because of this perspective, I view pornography as an institutional evil that preys on the disaffected, wounded and desperate members of society. I believe that even those who wholeheartedly embrace pornography's lie of sexual fulfillment and freedom (whether producers, actors or consumers) are still loved by God. Our calling as Christians is to examine ourselves and walk alongside those who have been damaged by this evil. We are not to demonize others, but to share God's healing, grace and mercy as they discover their identity in Christ. Healing and right thinking about our sexual nature are found in the person of Jesus Christ, Scripture, the power of the Holy Spirit and the ministry of the church.

Many excellent books have been written by Christian authors who explain in plain terms how men can deal with pornography. They use language common in Christian culture and easy for many men to grab hold of: lust of the flesh, sexual sin, diseased soul, sexual idolatry. Much good comes from using this language when wrestling with the reality of pornography. Many of these authors rightly frame pornography as more than just an ethical or legal matter—it is a *spiritual* matter.

Pornography is also a *physical* matter, rooted in the biological intricacies of our sexual design. In my opinion, nowhere is the complexity of our sexual nature seen more than in the wiring of the brain. Our reproductive organs are often given too much attention in the discussion of sexuality. It is the brain, however, where we feel the sexual longing, the arousal, the focus and the ecstasy that comes from sexual intimacy. Using spiritual and psychological language to describe the tenacious grip of sexually destructive patterns is helpful. But calls to pray harder, move the computer to the living room and get plugged into an accountability group only go so far. They come across as hollow to many men whose brains have been altered and rewired by their experiences with pornography. They have trained their brains to respond sexually to the pornography they consume.

We need to move to the next stage of dealing with pornography, cybersex addictions and sexual compulsions. We can find healthy ways to train the male brain to understand and act on its sexual nature. By appreciating our created nature and acknowledging pornography's unhealthy impact on our brain (and the rest of our body), we have a better path forward.

I hope that as recent scholarship in the brain sciences reframes and informs our ideas about how we are made, we can develop a better understanding of how fearfully and wonderfully made we are. Pornography taps into many men's wrong thinking about themselves, in places where their brains are most vulnerable to exploitation. But as we appreciate the reality of our sexuality and place it within the biblical narrative, we will see hope for redemption. As we more clearly see our need for redemption and the path of sanctification, we will be better equipped to heal from the wounds of pornography and allow our sexuality to be a necessary part of the process by which we are conformed to the image of Christ.

Part 1: How Pornography Works

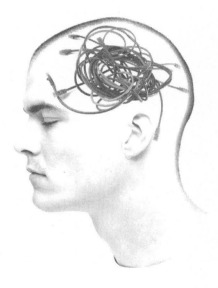

1

Saturated with Porn

PORNOGRAPHY IS DIFFICULT TO WRITE ABOUT for a variety of reasons. First, as a Christian, to even address it is to walk straight into the lion's den. I've received a mixture of odd glances and comments whenever I tell people that I am writing a book on pornography. "Oh, I get it . . . you're doing *research*. So do you look at it?" they ask. I find the jovial attitude some people have toward pornography disconcerting and disheartening. As a person of faith, I believe that pornography is a medium that degrades both men and women while offering the lie of on-demand sexual fulfillment, primarily to men. It is an industry that has saturated our culture and extends around the world. It is at the same time both an advertisement for sexual promiscuity and a product for consumption (Jensen et al., 1998; Jensen, 2007).

Pornography dishonors the image of God in an individual by treating him or her as a sexual object to be consumed directly or indirectly. Taking its name from the Greek terms *porne* and *graphein*, pornography is literally the writing about prostitutes (Paul, 2005). The current porn industry has capitalized on the commercialization of human sexuality as a commodity just as prostitution does.

Pornography takes human sexuality out of its natural context—intimacy between two human beings—and makes it a product to be bought and sold. By debasing the human body and valuing it in the same way we would something from the local convenience store, pornography promotes a human being's sexuality as a product for consumption. The product, another's sexuality, is evaluated through our own set of selfish needs. Which video, magazine or website will get me what I want with the maximum payoff? The pornographic selection may be consumed once, occasionally or on an ongoing basis, like a never-ending bottle of ketchup. When it no longer meets my sexual needs or fantasies, it can be thrown away. No need to recycle here. The law of supply and demand ensures there will always be another video, magazine or website.

Just as food is consumed and digested by the body, pornography is consumed by the senses and digested by the brain. In the digestive process, food is broken down so that it can supply the body with energy. Waste products are excreted to ensure the health of the organism. Similarly, pornography is taken into the brain via our senses, primarily through sight and touch. However, there is no process for the "waste" products associated with pornography to be removed. Pornography and our response to it alter our brain in a way that is difficult to undo. Pornography is the consumption of sexual poison that becomes part of the fabric of the mind.

PORNOGRAPHY AND THE FABRIC OF CULTURE

It should come as no surprise to anyone that pornography is big business. The estimated financial size of the worldwide sex industry is around $57 billion, with $12 billion (just over 20 percent) coming from the United States. While adult videos constitute the bulk of the porn industry, its tentacles are in many other media as well: magazines, escort services, strip clubs, phone sex, pay-per-view cable channels and adult content websites. It is significant that much of this industry is visual.

While there is debate about how big the adult entertainment industry actually is and how much money is generated by it, there is little doubt that the availability of pornography has dramatically increased over the past twenty-five years. With the advent of home video machines in the 1980s and the Internet in the 1990s, our culture has become saturated with sexually explicit and suggestive material. Porn has moved from seedy corner magazine stands and adult video stores to the privacy of our homes, offices and dorm rooms. The result is that pornography has crept into an astounding number of private lives. Because of its proliferation, the taboos that were once associated with it have been reduced or removed. Pornography today has become an accepted part of life for much of society.

I was recently listening to a sports radio talk show. The hosts abruptly switched from a discussion of Chicago sports teams to an invitation for callers to phone in with their nominations for the most creative "performance" names of adult film stars. Each of the hosts rattled off a number of risqué names without much hesitation. It was only a matter of minutes until their phone lines were jammed with callers chiming in with their favorites. The segment was immediately followed by one of their regular advertisers: a "gentleman's club." My guess is that this was not necessarily the result of any planning on the producer's part. The advertisements on the sports radio stations target their male audience just as powerfully as the billboards that I see whenever I drive to Chicago's O'Hare airport. Even in the isolation of our cars, the airwaves and skyline remind us that we are not free from the influence of the sex industry.

Many Christians find themselves in a cultural battle to protect both themselves and their children from this onslaught of sexual permissiveness. Pornography and the wider sex industry have brazenly walked through the front doors of the mass media into our televisions, computers and cell phones. See how long you can go without viewing or hearing something that has clear ties to the sex industry. The message is clear: Sex doesn't just sell—it is the motivation for living.

The movie *American Pie* has a number of sexually oriented scenes that are indicative of our cultural situation. In one scene, the main character is so desperate to see a pornographic movie that he vigilantly strains to make out the sexual images that have been distorted by a cable scrambler. His parents catch him masturbating to the warped images, and standard sophomoric humor ensues. In another scene the gawky father gives pornographic magazines to his son as a sort of rite of passage. Later, the young man webcasts his "seduction" of a foreign exchange student, with disastrous results.

I realize that *American Pie* is just a movie. It is not a documentary, and the director would probably say that it doesn't depict any actual events. But *American Pie* resonated with many young men, grossing over $235 million at the box office. Many young men can relate to the curiosity and magnetic power of the female form, the ritualistic introduction to pornography and the use of the Internet as a tool for sexual voyeurs.

In contrast, consider the outcry after the Janet Jackson breast-baring incident during the Super Bowl XXXVIII television halftime show in February of 2004. The 9/16th-of-a-second flash of her breast on television prompted thousands of angry letters to the Federal Communications Commission, which led to a fine being levied against CBS, an apology from Ms. Jackson and one of the highest Tivo replays on digital television recorders to date. The irony was that Ms. Jackson was for the most part fully clothed and that viewers had been exposed to numerous shots of cheerleaders gyrating in skin-tight pants. I wondered which was worse: an "accidental" glimpse of a bare breast or the lecherous, lingering "go-to-commercial" shots of NFL cheerleaders' cleavage?

What makes the outcry and the apology even more hollow is the lack of protest at the images of a near-naked Janet Jackson (and many other female celebrities) on the covers of music, celebrity and men's interest magazines over the past few years. The sexually titillating images are everywhere and relatively ignored. They have so subtly crept into the fabric of the culture that we have become desensitized and immune to them.

This influence of pornography is found on television as well. An episode of *Friends* details the addictive and mind-altering effects that free access to cable pornography has on Chandler and Joey. They refuse to let anyone turn off the television, lest their access be taken away. The following exchange shows pornography's effect on their perceptions of women:

Chandler: I was just at the bank and there was this really hot teller, and she didn't ask me to go do it with her in the vault! Joey: Same kind of thing happened to me! Woman pizza-delivery guy comes over, gives me the pizza, takes the money, and leaves! Chandler: What? No "Nice apartment, I bet the bedrooms are huge"? Joey: No! Nothing! Chandler: You know what? We have to turn off the porn.

Chandler and Joey both begin to believe that all women in real life are like the women in the pornography. Viewing porn changed their expectations of and interactions with women. While the episode is fictional, the impact of pornography on men's lives is very similar.

Whether it be strip clubs or prostitutes, Internet porn or phone sex lines, the sex industry preys on two sets of people: the consumers (the buyer) and the consumed (those involved in its production). Anyone who cruises pornographic websites, rents movies or buys magazines adds to the demand for pornography. Each website visit is used to recruit additional advertising monies and more content. Each video that is rented increases the demand for more releases. The consumer of pornography may not be doing anything illegal, but they add fuel to the inferno that is the sex industry. And sadly, it is fueled by the human souls who are involved in its production (Leahy, 2008).

EVALUATING PORNOGRAPHY

There are a number of ways that pornography can be evaluated. Some take an anecdotal approach—talking about it from their personal perspective, what they have seen, what they think about it, how it has affected them. Others discuss it within the context of society—an issue of free speech, a matter of censorship, political regulation, violence against women. Pornography can be construed as an art form, or as one of many avenues for the expression of sexuality in the media. Religious institutions have much to say about the morality of pornography. Many church groups have engaged it socially (like protests) and theologically (from the pulpit).

When you delve into the minefield of pornography research, a number of things become quickly apparent. The first is that there is an enormous volume of literature on the topic from any number of disciplines, including sociology, philosophy, theology, psychology and business. Few people have the time or expertise to be experts in all of these fields (I am not an exception to that rule). My training is in biopsychology, and the research in this area is scattered across journals ranging from urology to brain imaging to endocrinology.

The human being is an incredibly complex and beautiful creation, and our sexuality is one of the more complex aspects of who we are, not one of its simpler ones. But we are more than just sexual, reproducing animals. As a faculty member at a Christian liberal arts college, I have had the opportunity to explore the topic of theological anthropology. I have been enormously blessed by those who have thought deeply about what it means to be fully human. How are we created in God's image? What is our role in the story of creation? These questions are just as complex as those surrounding the functioning of our brains.

THE THREE DODGES

As I waded through the morass of published books and journal articles, I found a handful of scholars and clinical practitioners who have examined pornography and how it has infiltrated our culture. Jensen, Dines and Russo (Jensen et al., 1998) describe the Three Dodges as ways that many in the pornography debate try to obscure what pornography really is. These dodges confuse the issue by "dodging" and derailing any criticism of the industry or medium.

THE DEFINITION DODGE

What is pornography? How do you define the legal term "pornography"? Who decides what is pornographic?

The first dodge is all about semantics. At the core of the Definition

Dodge is the deflection of attempts to define in clear, straightforward terms what is pornographic. This dodge becomes a tool by which many avoid the topic. If you can't define it clearly, why bother getting upset about it? The Definition Dodge becomes a shield that many in favor of free access to porn hide behind by focusing narrowly on how to describe pornography. "What's pornography to you is art to me," they claim. Pornography is in the eye of the beholder.

Many argue that pornography is culturally defined and that culture changes. This line of reasoning is rooted in an ethical relativism that most college sophomores would be able to intellectually dismantle if inclined to do so. But this relativism is seductive. It becomes a convenient crutch whenever we are confronted with dilemmas that make us uncomfortable. The question of definition is a valid point, but the dodge relies on a moral and linguistic relativism that short-circuits any dialogue on the matter.

When any definition is provided, the conversation is redirected toward finding loopholes in the definition. Is pornography the depiction of a naked body? If that is the definition, we have to classify thousands of pieces of what are clearly art as pornography. Are there different levels of pornography? Where do you draw the line? And if you do draw a line, does it become a slippery slope? Rather than agreeing on a working definition, the goal of the Definition Dodge is to establish a roadblock so that the plain effects of pornography are never addressed.

In 1964, a landmark case ruled on by the United States Supreme Court offered one of the more memorable (and often ridiculed) examples of the Definition Dodge in action. An Ohio theater manager, Nico Jacobellis, appealed a state Supreme Court decision upholding his conviction and fine for showing a French film, *The Lovers*. The scene in question was a love scene that was controversial at the time. It would pale by today's standards and would probably be considered standard fare for many cable channels. In *Jacobellis v. Ohio*, Supreme Court Justice Potter Stewart addressed the difficulty of defining "hardcore pornography" within the context of a legal definition of *obscenity*. His comments are somewhat notorious.

> I shall not today attempt further to define the kinds of material I understand to be embraced within that shorthand description [hardcore pornography]; and perhaps I could never succeed in intelligibly doing so. But I know it when I see it, and the motion picture involved in this case is not that. (*Jacobellis v. Ohio*, 1964)

"I know it when I see it" has become a mocked phrase by pornography's advocates when dealing with a working definition of pornography. In a culture drifting into moral relativism, who decides what is pornographic? By this standard, pornography is offered as a form of art. Justice Stewart's remarks are echoed in C. S. Lewis's allegory *The Pilgrim's Regress* (Lewis, 1981). The protagonist, John, is held captive by the Spirit of the Age. John is given milk to drink, and after he extols the pleasant taste of the milk, the jailor who brought it to him chides him. Milk, he argues, is no different from any other substance that comes out of a cow's orifice, like dung, urine, vomit or sweat. John sighs and names his jailor as "a liar or only a fool, that you see no difference between that which Nature casts out as refuse and that which she stores up as food."

To a clearly ordered mind and conscience, the distinction between pornography and art is easily discernable if not readily definable. There is a clear difference between artistic nudity and the exploitation of the human form and sexuality. Those who wish to value artistic expression can ask a series of questions to distinguish pornography from true art.

1. How are women (and men) portrayed? Are they portrayed as people or objects to be lusted after?

2. How is sexual intimacy represented? Is it within a marital relationship or in isolation?

3. What is the purpose intended by the producer of the image (or media)?

4. What motivations do you (the viewer) bring to the exchange?

5. How explicit is the image? How much is left to the imagination?

Pornography inherently degrades and dehumanizes. Art celebrates the meaning and value of sexual intimacy between two individuals. In the exchange between artist and viewer in the artistic medium, it is important to consider the motives of the artist (producer) and the nature of the image. The artist wants to communicate a message or elicit an emotion from the audience. Gifted artists with pure motives can produce works of art that elicit powerful emotions or make profound statements. But regardless of one's motive and skill, the artist has a limited ability to control the motives of the audience.

In the most straightforward exchange, the artist's purposes are accomplished when an open audience receives the handiwork and responds as the artist intended. But this is not always the case. An artist can only do so much in creating a piece of art that celebrates the person depicted in it. A classic piece of art that is a nude can become a piece of pornography to a warped mind. Indeed a warped mind can make anything perverted. If the heart, mind and motives of the viewer are steeped in selfishness and perversion, even the greatest works of celebration can drive someone further into depravity. Consider the Song of Songs. It is an example of an erotic piece of literature with deep spiritual worth, but to a warped mind it can become a prelude to sexual fantasy and mental perversion.

Pornography is a medium where the intentions of the artist and the response of the viewer are just as important as the content of the medium. An artist may intend a portrait to be a celebration of beauty (i.e., a beautiful face), and the portrait may be nothing more than an oil-based representation of a woman's face. But if the image is viewed by someone who mentally ravages the person for his or her own purposes, valuing the self above the other, it can become pornographic.

PORNOGRAPHY DEFINED

Pornography is derived from the Greek word *porne*, which can be translated as "female captives" or "prostitutes." *Porneia* is often translated as "fornication," "whoredom" or "sexual immorality." In the New Testament there are twenty-six references to *porneia*. Of these twenty-six, six occur in Paul's letters to the Corinthians. The context of these letters is that believers are not to conform to the cultural norms that the church found itself confronted with. Our bodies are not made for *porneia* (1 Cor 6:13), we should run from it (1 Cor 6:18), we should not seek it out (1 Cor 7:2) and we should repent if we fall prey to it (2 Cor 12:21) (Bowring, 2005, p. 30).

In opposition to *porneia*, the apostle Paul offers an alternative: purity. For the Christian, purity is not limited to our sexual behavior but is the result of the process of sanctification. In his letter to the Philippians, Paul instructs, "Finally, brothers, whatever is true, whatever is honorable, whatever is just, whatever is pure, whatever is lovely, whatever is commendable, if there is any excellence, if there is anything worthy of praise, think about these things" (Phil 4:8). Purity is as much a matter of the mind as it is of the body, and it is important not to separate the two. The thoughts we think affect our body. The behaviors that we engage in affect our thinking. The interaction between thought and body is rooted in the neurobiology of the brain. Thoughts and behavior are woven together and intertwined with one another. This is how pornography and unhealthy sexuality pollutes the brain and the body together.

So what is pornography? Despite the difficulty in providing a definition that everyone can agree upon (because of the Definition Dodge), here are a few:

- The depiction of erotic behavior (as in pictures or writing) intended to cause sexual excitement. *(Merriam-Webster Dictionary)*

- Pornography is the material sold in the pornography shops for the purpose of producing sexual arousal for mostly male consumers. (Jensen et al., 1998)

- Sexually explicit pictures, writing, or other material whose primary purpose is to cause sexual arousal. *(American Heritage Dictionary)*

- Obscene writings, drawings, photographs, or the like, esp. those having little or no artistic merit. (Dictionary.com)

The *Catechism of the Catholic Church* addresses pornography as well:

2354 *Pornography* consists in removing real or simulated sexual acts from the intimacy of the partners, in order to display them deliberately to third parties. It offends against chastity because it perverts the conjugal act, the intimate giving of spouses to each other. It does grave injury to the dignity of its participants (actors, vendors, the public), since each one becomes an object of base pleasure and illicit profit for others. It immerses all who are involved in the illusion of a fantasy world. It is a grave offense. Civil authorities should prevent the production and distribution of pornographic materials.

For my money's worth, I prefer the definition put forward in the *Catechism*. Your choice might be another, but then again, that is at the core of the Definition Dodge.

THE CONSTITUTIONAL DODGE

With the Constitutional Dodge, pornography's proponents argue that the First Amendment of the U.S. Constitution protects the freedom to produce, market and distribute pornography in the context of free speech and free press. This appeals to our sense of independence and autonomy. Cries of "censorship" call out to the individualist in each of us, and the implied notion that we are not capable of responsible conduct rankles our pride. *Who makes the laws that say what grown men and women should be allowed to look at? Why should I trust them? Why do I need a law to tell me what I can and can't view?*

This dodge is another approach used to silence those who would speak against the porn industry. The Constitutional Dodge argues that pornographers are not producing material that is harmful, because all of their participants are consenting adults. They are merely meeting the market demand for sexually explicit material. Everyone is happy, so why legislate against it?

There are clear and obvious problems with this dodge. Some forms of pornography are already legislated against; the best example is child pornography. We do legislate what forms of pornography may be produced and consumed. Any retreat to a legal position which denies pornography's real-world effects on people—the emotional, social and psychological impact of pornography on the producers, participants and consumers both young and old—is nothing short of irresponsible. By highlighting the difficulties surrounding the passing and enforcing of reasonable legislative restrictions on pornographic material, the Constitutional Dodge prevents meaningful social discussion and misses the reality that pornography wounds its participants.

THE CAUSAL DODGE

Finally, for those of us in the research community, we run into difficulty with what may be referred to as the Causal Dodge. The technique behind this dodge is to highlight the limitations of research involving pornography. Today we live in a society that prefers its questions be answered by "scientific experts." However, the use of the scientific method becomes problematic when making ethical or legal statements about what to do with the results of these studies. Scientific theories are for making connections between variables, not determining their moral status. The Causal Dodge highlights this.

In most social and behavioral sciences there are three major approaches to studying a phenomenon. The first is a *descriptive* approach. With the descriptive approach, scientists attempt to objectively observe and describe what is present in the world. This approach uses case studies, surveys and naturalistic observation (just watching people). With this approach, a phenomenon is systematically described. The second approach is known as a *correlational* design. In correlational studies, researchers attempt to mathematically measure if the presence or absence of any one variable can reliably predict the presence or absence of another. For example: (1) do SAT scores reliably predict college GPA, or (2) does knowledge about a man's marital status provide any insight about his income? In a correlational design a relationship between two things is being established. One limitation of this design is the directionality of the relationship is undetermined. Consider our examples from above:

1. Do SAT scores reliably predict college GPA? It would appear that there is another variable (such as intelligence or scholastic aptitude) that is the underlying factor that causes both high SAT and high college GPA. Both of these tests might just be measuring the same causal variable (and this variable may be changing across time— intelligence increased with education, for example).

2. Does marital status provide any insight about a man's income? If we find that married men make more money than unmarried men, does that mean that getting married makes you a more stable person and thereby increases your performance at work (resulting in promotions) or that men who are better off financially attract women who are willing to marry them?

It becomes a "which came first, the chicken or the egg?" conundrum. Because of the limitations of how correlation research is conducted, you cannot make statements about the directionality (A causes B) of the variables measured. These types of causal statements are restricted to experimental approaches. Thus the Causal Dodge (or perhaps it should be called the Correlational/Causal Dodge) focuses narrowly on the limitations of correlational research in establishing causal relationships, deflecting criticism that pornography can have harmful effects.

The hallmark of *experimental* designs is manipulation of a variable (the causal or independent variable) by the researcher. This is followed by observation of the effects on another variable (the affected or dependent variable). Manipulating an independent variable and holding all other variables as constant as possible allows researchers to infer that any changes in the dependent variable are caused by differences in the independent variable. In this way, the direction of the relationship can be established (one variable is changed and changes in the other follow) and the majority of alternate (or confounding) explanations are minimized. The experimental approach gives greater confidence in saying that altering one variable causes a change in another.

The problem in much behavioral and social science research is that the experimental approach is often not feasible, nor is it ethical. To conduct a robust "experiment" on the developmental effects of pornography on children would require taking a number of individuals (let's say they are all genetic clones to minimize the effects of genetics), raising them under the exact same parenting conditions, minimizing their exposure to the outside world so that their life histories are as similar as possible, and then randomly assigning them into one of two groups. One group would be exposed to pornography and the other group prevented from seeing pornography (the independent variable). After a year we send them out into the world and see if there are any differences in any number of their behaviors (dependent variables). These might include porn-seeking behavior, attitudes toward women, sexual acts of violence, mental health issues or anything else porn might affect. Only under these types of conditions can you say that porn *causes* something else.

I hope the absurdity of this is apparent. If all of the current data regarding pornography is correlational and not causal, nothing can be definitively concluded about its impact, either negative or positive. This is at the heart of the Causal Dodge. The tobacco industry was able to hide behind this dodge for over fifty years. Smoking doesn't *cause* lung cancer because all of that research is correlational, right? It *may* cause lung cancer (as the Surgeon General's warning labels said), because it was *correlational* research, not experimental. Yet whenever there actually is a causal effect, a correlational relationship automatically follows. Sometimes it is true that where there is smoke, there is fire (pardon the pun).

The Causal Dodge worked for the tobacco industry for over fifty years, so it is not surprising that the porn industry has followed suit. The same argument is made. Because so little experimental research has been done on pornography and that much of what has been done is either descriptive or correlational, the issue is confused and the conclusion is drawn that pornography doesn't cause anything. The presence of correlations between exposure to pornography and a host of social, psychological, emotional and spiritual problems is the smoke. The ethical and practical limitations in proving there is a fire should not temporarily assuage us into a place where we deny that the fire exists. A better place to begin is to recognize that pornography is a significant contributing factor to many psychological and social ills.

THE THREE *AS* OF THE INTERNET

While many scholars may claim that modern pornography didn't really exist until the Victorian Era, it has been around for quite some time (Paul, 2005). Depictions of individuals engaging in sexual acts and materials that sexually arouse and titillate have been present for most of human history. But recent advances in the production, distribution and delivery of pornography have created such a realistic representation of sexual intercourse that it rivals the real thing.

> Like the Bible, the Internet is filled with tales of the transforming power of romantic love, as well as the destructiveness of misguided sexuality. People are people and are beset with yearnings, temptations, appetites, and lusts that have neither much changed, nor abated, over the millennia. . . . [H]umans have always faced sexual choices with the potential to lead them to decadence or transcendence. However, unlike the days of the Old Testament, the added element of computer technology makes modern times qualitatively different. (Cooper, 2002, pp. 1-2)

Pornography is often a driving force behind new technology, and it is no surprise that the Internet is the fertile soil where much pornography and pornography-related compulsions have their roots. The Three *As* of the Internet are accessibility, affordability and anonymity (Cooper, 2000). While the Three Dodges are used to prevent meaningful dialogue on the topic, the Three As address the reasons pornography has flourished online. These are the major reasons why the Internet has become such a powerful influence in the spread of pornography and the ease with which it has grabbed hold of so many men.

ACCESSIBILITY

Pornography is now much more accessible than ever before. Twenty years ago you needed to go to a specialty shop and actually interact with another human being to purchase a dirty magazine or rent a pornographic video. The prospect of someone seeing you purchase the material, cultural frowning upon of the pornography industry and the shame from being seen often produced enough fear to make many men avoid purchasing it altogether. These days, however, pornography is readily available on your computer, television or through mail order. You don't have to go into a shop to purchase it; it is only a few keystrokes and mouse clicks away.

AFFORDABILITY

Because of the ease of access, pornography is also much more affordable. In fact, a significant amount of online pornography is free. Many gateway sites offer free sample content, usually a small number of pictures or short video clips that are easily downloaded. These websites act as portals through which this free material is accessed without charge.

How do these sites stay online? Is it a pornographic version of altruism, maintaining a webpage at a person's individual expense to provide free material to the public? In some cases the answer is yes, but in most cases these sites receive advertising revenue from sponsors. These sponsors help keep these consolidated sample content sites in business for the express purpose of directing more traffic to their paid sites. The free samples can be fairly static (i.e., pictures, short video clips), but they whet the sexual appetite of the viewer and promise additional content for a fee. Those fees may not be exorbitant, but if a four-dollar fee for monthly access is paid by fifty thousand subscribers, that's a monthly revenue of $200,000. Portions of that are used to pay the gateway sites a modest advertising fee, and the remaining profit can be divided to procure additional material.

In a single day of shooting, three or four adult actors can film a number of sexual scenes that are easily prepared as still pictures, softcore and/or hardcore movies for both physical and online distribution. Production costs can be minimal, and amateur material lends to the feeling that "this could actually happen to me" or "these could be people in my neighborhood." This seeming reality serves to heighten the arousal in some men and appeals to a particular porn demographic. Combined with relatively affordable access to movie production equipment (complete with high-quality commercial cameras and video editing software) and inexpensive web hosting and programming, low-budget porn can be produced anywhere. It can be webcams set up for interactive sex chat or digital photography uploaded to a pay-for-access website. Porn is no longer manufactured and distributed only by technical experts in the San Fernando Valley, but in suburban and rural communities across the country.

ANONYMITY

People hide their porn habits and try to make sure that no one else finds out. Porn users put as many barriers as possible between themselves and others so that plausible deniability can always be maintained. Anonymous online technologies contribute to this cycle of secrecy.

If you are sitting alone in your home accessing porn in private, no one knows who you are. You don't have to go out and run the risk of someone actually seeing you purchase it. The use of porn on the Internet has increased in an astounding fashion in the past ten or fifteen years. The social stigma associated with watching porn has diminished over the years, and any remaining shame is easily addressed by hiding in the confines of a dorm room, bedroom, office or den. Your service provider might monitor which sites you are viewing, but even then your identity is relatively anonymous. You can change your online identity and pretend to be someone else.

Anonymity can also lead to hyperpersonal relationships online. Freed from any prospect of accountability and the absence of a real person in front of them, the anonymity available online leads some men to relate differently with other anonymous partners than they do with people in real life. They reveal things about themselves that they normally would not, increasing the likelihood of engaging in risky behavior.

THE TRIPLE-C ENGINE

In his book *Sex and the Internet: A Guide for Clinicians*, clinical psychologist Al Cooper (Cooper, 2002) explores the notion that the Internet is driven by what he calls the "Triple-C Engine." The Internet is not a static, passive medium for the viewer, but one in which people can interact with the content. They are not merely passive consumers of the pornographic content, but the technology allows them to become potential senders in the process. They can *communicate* and *collaborate* as active members of a *community*.

Communication. Communication provides opportunities to share our lives with others. This is an important part of being human— telling your story and letting others know who you are. Today this can take place through electronic communication such as text messaging or connecting via webcam. Interacting with others reinforces the fact that others are acknowledging and responding to you. Why do we do it? Because it allows us to share our lives with others, despite the artificial nature of the interaction.

The ability to communicate with others through the Internet extends into pornography and makes it interactive. Porn need not be just a snapshot of nakedness or a sexual act that was recorded in the past, but it can be dynamic cybersexuality, communicating in real time. Men can webchat with a model on the other end and ask her to perform specific acts. Our sexuality is meant to be an embodied mutual exchange between husband and wife as they discover God's love. Instead, the Internet serves as the relational medium in which sexual arousal and stimulation are channeled, and it operates as the communicative mediator in the expression of our sexuality.

Collaboration. A second engine, collaboration, allows people to work together toward a goal. One of the great benefits of the Internet is that it allows people who are separated by distance to interact with each other. But the Internet has also enabled the collection of warehouses of digital porn, the establishment of cyberprostitution and networks of illicit sexual materials. The collaborative nature of the Internet has allowed people to exercise their sexual brokenness, such as file sharing of digital child pornography libraries.

From a social perspective, once you start engaging in cybersexual behavior, you move from communication with other users of pornography to collaboration with one another. It develops from "Hey, check this out" (communication) to "Let's get together and start making something" (collaboration). And whenever you collaborate, you begin establishing community.

Community. Those collectively sharing their lives with each other and working toward common goals will form a community (Rheingold, 2000). Those who share their porn with each other think of each other as fellow members in their social network. They share common interests, passions and characteristics. They follow certain rules about how they interact with each other and think of themselves as part of a larger group. As members of the community, they share with each other, participate with each other and even work toward meeting each other's needs. Given the needs for connection and sexual expression that the Internet and pornography imperfectly meet, the logical outcome is that of a community of people who are bound together by the common bond of pornography.

THE PERFECT STORM

It is not the shouting of pornography that gives it so much power over men. It is the whispering of the lie of sexual fulfillment that prey on our human insecurities. When men believe those lies, they develop psychological and behavioral habits that prevent relational fulfillment. Pornography shapes and rewires us in such a way that we become unable to see women as we should. We no longer direct our sexual drives in appropriate ways. Porn narrows our ability to live a good and holy life.

In her article "The Porn Myth," feminist Naomi Wolf argues that pornography has moved into the mainstream of the cultural arena, and in large part due to the Internet, it has "pornographized" our culture. She observes that many feminists were wrong in their assumption that pornography would turn men into raving sexual beasts bent on all forms of sexual mayhem. Instead, she argues, over the years the pervasiveness of pornography has rendered men less sexually responsive to real women.

I believe she is right. Pornography has numbed the healthy sexuality of men who are active consumers of it. Wolf writes,

> For most of human history, the erotic images have been reflections of, or celebrations of, or substitutes for, real naked women. For the first time in human history, the images' power and allure have supplanted that of real naked women. Today, real naked women are just bad porn. (Wolf, 2003)

So how did we get to this perfect storm of cultural, technological and psychological factors converging on so many men? How has pornography been able to hijack lives and blunt the expression of healthy sexuality? How should the Christian church respond to the current state of affairs? We need to see just how pornography corrupts us to our core. We need to go back and reexamine what it means to human—to be created in the image of God. We need to understand what it means to be created male. We need to have a theology that understands the importance of our sexuality and what this looks like for men. And we need to respond in a way that honors those who have been affected by pornography and to help in restoration, redemption and healing.

REFERENCES

Jacobellis v. Ohio. 1964. 378 U.S. 184.

Bowring, Lyndon, ed. 2005. *Searching for intimacy.* Waynesboro, GA: Authentic Media.

Catechism of the Catholic Church—English translation. 1997. (2nd Ed.). U.S. Catholic Conference, Inc.

Cooper, Al. 2000. *Cybersex: The dark side of the force.* Philadelphia: Brunner-Routledge.

Cooper, Al. 2002. *Sex and the internet: A guidebook for clinicians.* New York: Brunner-Routledge.

Jensen, R., G. Dines and A. Russo. 1998. *Pornography: The production and consumption of inequality.* New York: Routledge.

Jensen, Robert. 2007. *Getting off: Pornography and the end of masculinity.* Cambridge, MA: South End Press.

Leahy, Michael. 2008. *Porn nation.* Chicago, IL: Northfield Publishing.

Lewis, C. S. 1981. *The pilgrim's regress: An allegorical apology for Christianity, reason and romanticism.* Grand Rapids, MI: Eerdmans.

Paul, P. 2005. *Pornified: How pornography is transforming our lives, our relationships, and our families.* New York: Times Books.

"Pornography." Dictionary.com <http://dictionary.reference.com/browse/pornography>.

"Pornography." Merriam Webster Online Dictionary. <www.merriam-webster.com/dictionary/pornography>.

Rheingold, H. 2000. *The virtual community: Homesteading on the electronic frontier.* Cambridge, MA: MIT Press.

Wolf, N. 2003. The porn myth. *New York Magazine* 20.

2

The Corruption of Intimacy

"Of all these assumptions, however, none has been more deeply ingrained than the belief that physically attractive women's bodies are the most magnificent spectacles in nature and that men are destined to fervently desire them, to compete for them, to sacrifice emotional and physical well-being for them, but rarely to enjoy them except from afar."

GARY R. BROOKS, *THE CENTERFOLD SYNDROME*

"IS PORN A SIN?" THIS IS ONE OF THE FIRST QUESTIONS that I am regularly asked by both Christians and non-believers. Most of the time the person isn't interested in knowing about pornography's virtue. It merely serves as the tip of the iceberg for a question closer to the heart. For some, the question is one that is asked through a religious filter. The use of the word "sin" as opposed to alternate terms such as "wrong," "bad," "dangerous" or "unhealthy" places the conversation solidly in the realm of theology. They want to use the terms "evil" or "sinful." Many in the religious community already have the answer to their question, and they are just testing to see if I am going to back them up or if I am some sort of liberal heretic. Any answer other than, "Yes, pornography is a sin," and I run the risk of losing any religious credibility that comes with my position as a professor at a Christian college.

But for the person who views sexuality as being an integral part of their religious system, it is the right and proper question to ask. It recognizes that sexual intimacy is a significant dimension of our createdness and has an inherent meaning that transcends the mechanics of reproduction. It fits within a larger theology of our finitude. The need for sustenance, water, shelter and contact is a constant reminder that our physical needs are mere shadows of the deeper spiritual needs that can only be met by our Creator.

For others, the question "Is porn a sin?" is still rooted in the religious realm, but it is a deeper, much more personal question. It is not directed at broad systematic theology or carving out the correct dogmatic niche in a religious framework. For these individuals, the question is rooted in a fear that they have polluted themselves and are beyond spiritual restoration. In short, they are convinced that because they have looked at porn or have an ongoing relationship with it, they are going to be condemned to hell. Their history of repeated consumption of porn has become such a shameful part of their existence that they ask the question, holding out for some shred of hope, some lifeline to be thrown by a so-called "expert," that they are not forever lost to the pits of hell.

Some may be perfectly inclined to leave the question as a religious one, but others are bent on arguing against any religious restrictions against sexuality. It is an anti-religious spirit that asks for (or goads) a response. "Is porn as sin?" they ask, hoping for an affirmative response. An answer of "yes" becomes an invitation to deride anyone who would hold that human sexuality is anything other than an animalistic need that has no moral or religious meaning. Sex is just sex; any attempt to add onto it religious significance is out of place. This view holds the hedonistic pleasure principle above any moral or religious objections to pornography. It encourages us to maximize our orgasmic experiences and shrug off all the unnecessary guilt and shame that prudish religious types try to laden you with. Besides, they point out, everyone does it—even the religious types. The numerous religious figures who have failed to uphold the sexual ethics they preach are hypocrites at the highest level. The underlying goal is not to justify pornography, but to mock and tear down the religious systems that would consider the sexual act as having a transcendent meaning.

A MORAL QUESTION

Pornography need not be restricted to religious discussions. Many look at the effects that pornography has on individuals or its impact as part of the sociological landscape. Their question may be more properly phrased, "Is pornography bad, damaging or dangerous to our society?" One need only look at the major cultural, technological, psychological, biological and spiritual factors converging in our world today to see how pornography has become one of the trademark corruptions of humanity. The fact that our culture is dedicated to capitalism and consumerism contributes to one of the age-old advertising mantras, "Sex sells." Nearly half a century after the sexual revolution of the 1960s, we are still experiencing its aftershocks (Paul, 2005).

Men share with women the same basic needs of humanity. The need for intimacy, to be known and to know, to be close, affirmed, loved; all are human needs. The need for intimacy requires that we understand who we are and share that with those we long to be known by. As we become more intimate, the other speaks into us things about ourselves that we could not possibly know from the inside. We allow the one we are intimate with to discover us in ways we could not do on our own, and we do so with them. It is a process that develops and deepens over time. We know ourselves more fully because we are known more fully. The intimacy that we have with God and with others enables us to move along the journey toward either sanctification or depravity.

Pornography corrupts the ability to be intimate. It pulls consumers and producers in with the promise of intimacy, but fails to deliver the connection between two human beings (Balswick and Balswick, 1999; Kelsey and Kelsey, 1999).

THE ATTRACTION

Something about pornography pulls and pushes at the male soul. The pull is easy to identify. The naked female form can be hypnotizing. A woman's willingness to participate in a sexual act or to expose her nakedness is alluring to men. The awareness of one's own sexuality, the longing to know, to experience something as good wells up from deep within. An image begins to pick up steam the longer we look upon it. It gains momentum and can reach a point where it feels like a tractor-trailer rolling downhill with no brakes.

And that is just the naked form. The more dynamic and lifelike the pornography (i.e., videos, interactive cybersex), the greater the neurological and hormonal tsunami it initiates. This tsunami can overwhelm your ability to make wise decisions (Seymour and Dolan, 2008, pp. 662-71; Ariely and Loewenstein, 2006, p. 87; Schwarz, 2000, pp. 433-40). The images and videos bring you to a window in time where you can cheat reality. This alternate reality has few immediate consequences except for the promise of sexual arousal and orgasm. The knowledge and promise of the transcendent sexual ecstasy that is waiting can be overwhelming. When caught in the spiraling psychological and physiological pull of pornography, the prospect of escaping it is unpleasant. You want to let it pull you in.

Many men can spend hours looking at pornography, continually increasing their sexual arousal and tricking themselves into preparing for a sexual encounter with another person that doesn't (usually) happen. As they do, they are neurologically training themselves to respond to the type of images they view. It is not just the actual visualization of the naked form, but it is the mental manipulation and fantasy that increases the need for a partner in intimacy. Men see many sexual cues throughout the day, but they also mentally manipulate these images and fantasize about what it might be like to have intercourse with one of these women. The way that a male brain is organized in being one-track, goal-oriented and visuospatial (mentally manipulating objects) make it the perfect playground for sexual fantasy—the mental consumption of another's sexuality (Loftus, 2002).

Because of these cognitive structures and the ability to store sexual images that are associated with sexual arousal and gratification, the minds of many men become hidden, personalized adult film studios. Any women they have seen and anyone else they can imagine are their performers. As porn and fantasy take control of the mind, it becomes a dream theater that is transposed over the waking world. Every woman they come into contact with is objectified, undressed and evaluated as a willing (or unwilling) mental sexual partner. She is rated on her imagined sexual proficiency and then either stored for later use or discarded as worthless. This mental consumption of a person is a violation of the image of God in each of us.

Many women can tell when a man is mentally undressing them. My students report how uncomfortable this makes them feel when they know it is being done. Women in my classes often speak up when we discuss this and share their unease. One female student said, "I can tell when a guy is mentally using me as a plaything in his head, even when he is talking to me. He doesn't look into my eyes. He fidgets. He keeps looking at my [breasts] and he thinks I don't notice, but I do. It takes everything in me to keep from screaming. When a guy does that to me, I just want to go home and take a shower."

It's not that they don't want to be seen as sexual—they do. Most of us do; it's part of being human and our longing for intimacy. They just don't want to look in the face of a man they are trying to have a conversation with and see themselves reflected back as a sexual consumable. I am impressed with the ability of many women to detect when this is occurring in a conversation with a man. Not only do these women walk away with a negative impression of the man they were talking to, these women also say that the mental undressing and manipulation leaves them with a feeling of sexual uncleanliness.

THE AVOIDANT PUSH

In contrast to the attraction of pornography, part of our nature pushes against it. The arousal that it produces can also have an element of fear, revulsion or a need to avoid it. While many men indulge freely without any notion of restraint, others are repulsed by their response to pornography. The arousal that they experience sexually is accompanied by a conflicting sense of shame, guilt and/ or anxiety. Such men have a sense that something is just not right about what they are doing.

The nagging voice is repressed while viewing pornography, but afterward there is a gnawing sense that we shouldn't have looked. We intuitively know that what we saw was not meant for us. We have intruded into someone's intimate space. To the properly oriented conscience, viewing pornography elicits a healthy sense of guilt. To the seared conscience, one that has been ground down by abuse, fear, selfishness or repeated exposure to sin, pornography is just something you do. The seared conscience is forced either to turn against itself and plunge into the despair of self-loathing and unhealthy shame or to adopt new standards that allow for the acceptability of pornography. That standard may work for a time, but ultimately it leads to hurt, pain and suffering.

The unfortunate truth is that much of the pain resulting from pornography may be in the lives of others rather than the one with the seared conscience. Marriages, families, friendships, careers and ministries are often destroyed by the effects of pornography on a man.

FIRST CONTACT

During my childhood, I knew a boy named Max. He was an only child, raised by his divorced mother. His father was not in the picture most of the time, and Max wrestled with the sense of abandonment and guilt common to many children of divorce. On a weekend trip to his father's house when he was twelve, he came across some copies of *Playboy* and, not surprisingly, was sexually aroused. His father's stash of pornography was sufficiently large that Max took a chance that one magazine wouldn't be missed. He selected a magazine with a cover model that he found particularly attractive and packed it in his bag. The rest of the weekend he was incredibly anxious. He couldn't wait to get back to his home so that he could look at the magazine. He was especially nervous that his father might find out about his newfound interest and was very relieved when the weekend visit was over.

Once he was home, Max rushed to his room and hid the magazine in a place that he was relatively certain his mother wouldn't find. Max then began to experience a new wave of anxiety. He was certain that his mother would not approve of the magazine, and he did not want to deal with her religious faith. Max knew that stealing the magazine was wrong, but he also knew that he couldn't help himself. He just had to look at the pictures, but only when it was safe.

Max lay awake most of the night with the magazine and the guilt fresh on his mind. He was fearful that his mother would wake up if he got out of bed to get the magazine, but he couldn't get it out of his mind. He finally fell asleep late that night and rose the next morning tired and distracted. He went to school and socialized with his friends, but was reluctant to share what he had done. He rushed home after school knowing that his mother would not get home from work for another hour. Once home, he pulled the magazine from its hiding place and began to scan each page, unable to take his eyes off of the pictures. He recalled, "It was like I was taking in these images, and they created a feeling inside me that I had never had before. It was kind of like having a crush on a girl or wanting to kiss her, but there was this growing pressure down under my stomach that I didn't know what to do with. I felt like I was going to explode."

Max hid the magazine and went to school the next day. When he got home later that afternoon, he checked the hiding place to steal a quick glimpse while his mother was making dinner. The magazine wasn't there! Max knew that his mom must have found it and taken it. He was terrified. When he went down to dinner, his mother didn't speak to him and glared at him as he ate. He sat through dinner in uncomfortable silence. When he went back to his room, he cried. He wondered if his mom thought his dad had given it to him. He didn't want her to stop his visits to his dad's place. He wished he had his dad or a big brother who could explain it all to him, and he was ashamed of what his mother must have thought about him.

Many men can relate to Max's story. It is an example of the mingling of excitement, anxiety, shame and confusion that often accompanies a boy's first exposure to pornography. Max's experience, however, is not representative of first-time exposure for most boys today. While softcore pornographic magazines may have been the norm for "first contact" prior to the 1990s, today first contact primarily happens through the Internet, with images ranging all over the pornography spectrum. The emotions experienced by Max, however, still ring true in the youth of today.

HEALTHY VS. UNHEALTHY SEXUALITY

What is healthy sexuality and how can it be contrasted with unhealthy sexuality? Let's consider the following distinctions (Maltz and Maltz, 2008).

Many of the men struggling with pornography that I have worked with have shared how frustrated and ashamed they are at their automatic response to the women they meet. Their eyes are immediately drawn to the woman's breasts, buttocks or hips. This objectifying of women, looking at their "parts" and evaluating them as potential sexual partners has become reflexive, a consequence of their habitual use of pornography and preoccupation with their own sexual fantasies. One of the greatest victories that a man recovering from an addiction to pornography and compulsive sexual acting out has is when he can look at a beautiful woman and not feel the need to mentally treat her as a sex object.

A man with a properly oriented conscience and filled with the Spirit has a healthy view of sexuality. He values the image of God in the women (and men) that he meets and has trained his mind to take these sexual thoughts captive. He is able to experience great freedom in his interactions with women. He does not mentally bed every woman he meets. Being able to see a woman as a human being and not a sexual plaything is a critical step for the man recovering from pornography dependence toward sanctification. But for the man who is caught in the grips of pornography, all women are potential sexual

Table 2.1. Healthy Sexuality vs. Unhealthy Sexuality (Modified from Maltz & Maltz, 2008, p. 182)

Godly/Healthy Sexuality	Pornography/Unhealthy Sexuality
Caring	Using
Sharing with someone	"Doing to" someone
Honoring	Shameful
Authentic	Deceitful
Enhances your identity	Compromises your identity
Emotional bonding	Emotional separateness
Spiritual unity	Spiritual separateness
Morally saturated	Free of moral convention
Communication is essential	Communication is optional
Other-directed	Selfish, self-directed
Biblical boundaries	Has no limits
Involves all of the person	Is visual and genital
Naturally drives us toward intimacy	Unnaturally drives us toward compulsions
Naturally drives toward sanctification	Unnaturally drives toward depravity
Matures into responsible habits	Escalates toward irresponsible risks
Nurtures the spouse	Hurts the partner
Is an expression of love	Is an expression of usefulness
Humanizes	Objectifies
Honors the image/imaging of God in you	Dishonors the image/imaging of God in you
Honors the image/imaging of God in spouse	Dishonors the image/imaging of God in another
Provides emotional, moral, psychological and relational clarity	Produces emotional, moral, psychological and relational confusion

partners. He thinks this because that is what pornography has taught him. It is impossible to view pornography and not have it affect one's belief about women.

So how do men respond to the confusion produced by pornography and unhealthy practices of sexually acting out? Many employ common cognitive defense strategies. Viewing porn can be denied, minimized, normalized, rationalized or even celebrated.

DENIAL

Doing research on pornography viewing is difficult not because there are insufficient materials or participants. It is because many men when asked will flat out deny that they regularly view pornography. "Sure," they may say, "I've looked at it in the past, but I don't any more." Many men admit to regularly viewing pornography only under the conditions of anonymity and confidentiality. Face-to-face surveys consistently show lower rates of pornography viewing when compared to online surveys that do not require the answer be given directly to another person. This is not uncommon when dealing with issues that carry a cultural stigma. Many men do not want to disclose their viewing of pornography even though there is a cultural trend toward accepting (and even celebrating) it. The potential stigma that comes along with viewing pornography is too much to risk for honest disclosure.

Some men may deny that they view pornography because they have equated the term "pornography" with graphic, violent or sexually explicit materials and place "softcore" pornography (pictures of naked women or videos of sexual acts that do not show the genitalia) in the "non-pornography" category. They would be better described as "softcore" porn users, but porn users nonetheless. Whether it is by being conveniently forgetful, performing some definitional gymnastics or being downright dishonest, many men deny that they view pornography. In these instances, it is difficult to discover the impact of pornography because of the lack of disclosure.

The lack of honesty with respect to porn participation is problematic. However, we should not assume that everyone who says they don't look at porn is lying. Those who don't use or seek out pornography regularly have learned appropriate ways to allow their sexual drive to direct them toward intimacy and sanctification. But for those who haven't learned to be honest about their use of pornography, other warning signs may indicate their involvement. We can only warn that all sin will eventually come to light and that confession and repentance are necessary to start on the path toward healing. This stage can often be the most problematic for men to pass through. As is the case with all habitual problems and addictions, it is important to get out of the denial phase before any healing can take place.

MINIMIZATION

"Well, I do look at porn, but only occasionally. It's not like I'm addicted to it or anything." For the user of pornography who admits that he regularly views material and acts out in response to it, the next appeal is often to try and make it appear minimal. They argue that their pornography use is insignificant and has no real effect on their life. Often using vague statements and refusing to offer details, men will try to minimize the amount of porn they use, the frequency at which they do and the effects of it on their life as inconsequential. When their conscience requires them to answer affirmatively and they feel there is a certain amount of safety in doing so, they will underreport their involvement. Once again, not everyone who reports minimal viewing of pornography is lying, but in some cases, minimization is a prelude to the next step in the process.

NORMALIZATION

Some men who have gone beyond denial and minimization in their use of porn offer the excuse, "Everybody does it." Explaining the use of pornography as a common form of entertainment is referred to as normalization. In normalization, the appeal shifts from treating porn as if it is something that shouldn't be done (as in denial or minimization) to an acceptable behavior. The normalization of viewing pornography moves it away from being a bad thing to instead being an expected behavior. No longer is it something to be hidden, but it becomes a standard of conformity to cultural rules. It also is offered as a sign that the viewer is *normal*. To not view porn, with this line of thinking, is to be abnormal. Not viewing porn would mean you are unhealthy. But repeated exposure to pornography leads to desensitization and acceptance of things that should not be accepted.

The problem with appeals to cultural norms is that these norms are constantly in flux. Viewing pornography and sexually acting out to it was not the norm fifty or one hundred years ago. Just because something is a cultural norm does not make it morally right or wrong, good or evil. For the Christian, the moral standing of an action is governed by Scripture and principles that are in line with the character of God. Our sexuality is one of the strongest forms of intimacy through which God reveals himself as love. Scripture teaches that our sexual relationships should be reserved for a man and a woman in the exclusive covenant of marriage.

RATIONALIZATION AND JUSTIFICATION

Some users and producers of pornography argue that there are clear social and economic reasons for the production and consumption of pornography. Rationalization is the use of a logical argument to give permission *prior to* the viewing of pornography or acting out. Justification is the use of a logical argument to excuse viewing of pornography or acting out *after* the fact. You rationalize what *you are going to do* and you justify *what you just did*. Men using these approaches might rationalize or justify that using pornography provides a sexual outlet for someone when their partner is not willing or for those who don't have partners. It may be a means through which a single person can have their sexual needs met, or a way to avoid sexually transmitted diseases (STDs). Some therapists would argue that it can teach sexual technique or be used as a therapeutic tool to bring partners closer together. Many producers of pornography argue that they are providing a product to consumers and that if they didn't, those consumers might act out inappropriately.

I once read an article in which an adult movie actor suggested that the industry should be lauded because it provides a means for uneducated and unintelligent female performers to make a lavish wage. The participants are engaging in consensual sex and actually getting paid for it (an appeal that is not surprisingly similar to that offered for the legalization of prostitution). Many men jump on board with this argument and appealing to standards of lower moral value to justify the use and production of pornography. It distracts from the heart of the matter, which is that human beings are being manipulated to use their sexuality for a purpose other than that which it was intended for—intimacy. By making the sexual act about pleasure or profit, we lose sight of the fact that these things are secondary to the primary purpose of our sexuality.

CELEBRATION

Over time and with repeated exposure, many men so completely buy into the lies that pornography sells that they do not even feel a need to defend their habits. They have so lost the ability to see women portrayed as human beings. They embrace the horror of sexual exploitation and celebrate their addiction to it. They speak openly about their favorite performers and their collections. Having passed through the stages of normalization and rationalization, they have lost all moral and ethical reservations about its place in society and its damaging effects on their own relationships. In their mind, the world would be a better place if everyone just got over their puritan, antiquated views on human sexuality. They see pornography as the logical and preferred outcome of our male biology, female usefulness and our current media and technology.

We celebrate the things that we hold in high esteem. We celebrate marriages, anniversaries, birthdays, graduations and holidays. We celebrate the achievements of others, the life of those who have lived well, or the accomplishment of a worthy task. But when a person gets to the place where they celebrate the exploitation of women's and men's bodies for their own sexual gratification, the conscience is seared and the moral compass of the man has become seriously compromised.

This celebration can sometimes result in a rather strange manifestation of the objectification of women (and pornographic material) known as trophyism. Trophyism is the mentality whereby a man thinks of his sexuality as a contest against other men with the sexual domination of women and orgasm as the prizes. The roots of trophyism begin early and are seen in sexual conquests such as the first to get to "first base," the first to lose his virginity or the one to sleep with (and perhaps marry, but not necessarily) the most beautiful, sexually attractive woman. All of these "conquests" contribute to an objectified view of women.

I remember chatting with one man who was so proud of his porn collection that he beamed as he described it. "They're all awesome. You can borrow whatever you want," he told me, "but make sure you get them back to me as soon as possible. I don't like having my women cheat on me." His remarks seemed ridiculous given that there were probably thousands of the same videos circulating throughout the country. The innuendo that I would masturbate to them suggested that it would be the same as actually having sex with them. But he saw the performers as ultimately his own—his possessions. The images could be loaned, but at the end of the day they were to be returned. The fact that the performers were not real was dissonant with his hoarding behavior. Viewing the women and their images as his was a sign of his manliness. Unfortunately, the pornography and his view of women impaired his ability to have a real relationship with a real woman. He was so concerned about the fidelity of his female video performers that he was unable to be intimate or faithful to a real woman.

CORRUPTING INTIMACY

Many social factors have played into the explosive growth of pornography in Western culture. Corporate, technological and industrial changes over the past 150 years have isolated us and disrupted much of how our understanding of masculinity and sexuality are passed from generation to generation. We have become an increasingly individualistic society that elevates the power of the individual over the worth of others. The sexual revolution ushered in a sense of sexual entitlement that offered the promise of sexual transcendence, yet delivered increased promiscuity and decreased intimacy.

The increasing political polarization over the past twenty years has framed pornography as a cultural war between sexually repressed, mindless religious fanatics and progressive, orgasmic, freed sexual liberals. The rapid growth in the use and availability of media technology has given pornography wide exposure. Factor into the equation confusion about what it means to be a man and the biological predispositions of the male brain and you have the perfect storm for pornography and cybersexual compulsions, addictions and impulse control disorders.

The experience of sexual intimacy is properly intended between a husband and wife in a maturing healthy relationship. When pornography is acted upon, sexual technique replaces sexual intimacy. In the absence of a meaningful, relational context, nearly all of the elements of truly meaningful sexual intimacy are absent. Pornography teaches its students to focus on the physiology of sexual sensations and not on the relationships for which those sensations are intended.

Many men feel a deep sense of *shame* as a result of viewing and sexually acting out to pornography. Shame can be internal disappointment with ourselves or can be placed on us by a wider community. It is an attempt to cover up a sense of unworthiness or agonizing vulnerability. It involves exposure and judgment, with resulting feelings of insufficiency, defectiveness, inadequacy or unworthiness. At the core of shame is the belief that the individual is not worthy of love. In some cultural contexts shame is used to motivate others to change their behavior. This shame comes from the outside, imposed on us by our culture, community or family. But it can also come from within, imposed on us after a sense of guilt has been warped into a denial of our worth, value and identity in Christ.

It is critically important to recognize the difference between shame and guilt. Guilt is the feeling that we get when we do something that our conscience tells us is wrong. This conscience, our internal moral compass, serves as protection for both ourselves and for those around us. When our actions or thoughts have led to a violation or injury of another person, guilt can be a good emotion. It is a guide that can make us aware of when we have injured others. Healthy responses to guilt are confession, repentance, forgiveness and restoration.

Sometimes there is a gray area between guilt and shame. A person can know he is "guilty" but have no emotional response to the guilt. Oftentimes this is a person with a seared conscience. These individuals, at the extremes, can become sociopaths. But everyone has the capacity to know that they did something wrong yet find ways to excuse it, minimize it or even enjoy it.

The problem with shame is that it is based on more than just what we do. While guilt is primarily based on our actions, shame is based more on our belief about ourselves. The severity of our sense of guilt can sometimes lead us to a place where we feel a sense of shame. As we identify with those whom we have injured, we move from a healthy sense of guilt into a warped understanding of forgiveness, grace and mercy. It is here that many debate whether or not shame is God-given. Some argue that there are logical grounds for people feeling shame or for the culture to shame someone.

It is common in some traditions for a person to be publicly shamed as a way of punishing them for some transgression or attempting to motivate them toward a more pious life. Others argue that shame is rooted in a person's belief about themselves. All people were created in the image of God. To have a view of oneself that is rooted in unworthiness dishonors the image of God intrinsic in every individual. My belief is that all shame is unhealthy because it denies the intrinsic worth and value that God places on each human being. God does not call us to a life of shame but to a life of freedom as we move from awareness of our sinfulness to confession and repentance, to redemption and healing, to ministry and sanctification. Shame only offers the lie of worthlessness, and a sense of worthlessness creates fertile soil for the continued exercising of sexual brokenness.

Sexual shame finds a unique place in humanity. Because of the taboos on sexuality that are found in many cultures and the reality that our sexuality is a foundational part of what makes a person human, sexual shame undercuts a person's sense of worth, value and identity. Actions that have been done to someone (such as rape or incest) can also violate a person's sense of self. Actions that someone does to another sexually (such as sexual coercion or solicitation of a prostitute) can scar the victim as well as the perpetrator. This can lead to a strong yet unhealthy connection between the two.

The lie that pornography can somehow enhance intimacy is seductive. Even if a husband and wife view pornography together, they are intruding on the sexual intimacy, however fraudulent, of others. The sharing of sexual intimacy between a husband and wife should not be a public act.

> The myth about porn is that it frees the libido and gives men an outlet for sexual expression which liberates mind and body. This is truly a myth. I have found that pornography not only does not liberate men but on the contrary is a source of bondage. Men masturbate to pornography only to become addicted to the fantasy. There is no liberation for men in pornography. (U.S. Attorney General's commission on pornography, 1986, p. 1)

When men realize that they have bought a lie and that it has failed to deliver on its promise of intimacy, they become imprisoned by shame. They intuitively know that they need true intimacy, but they are incapable of having it when they are in isolation from real relationships with real people.

Another lie is that the most important thing in life is sexual gratification. If you are not being sexually gratified as frequently as possible with as many partners as possible, you are somehow being deprived of a life that is worth living. This sense of deprivation is a key factor that leads many men into depression and leaves them with a sense of hopelessness. The fixation on sexual gratification becomes so pronounced that they develop tunnel vision in other areas of their lives. Ironically, development of these neglected areas—their personality, spirituality and creative energies—would help them find a greater sense of accomplishment and meaning in their lives. Because they neglect these other areas, they spiral downward into depression and isolation. Their shame increases and they become frantic, looking for a way out. But all they have is a relationship to porn, which they turn to again and again, only to be continually disappointed. The cyclical nature of this process increases their shame.

Pornography reduces the worth of the partner to nothing more than an object to be penetrated for personal pleasure (Jensen, 2007). It acts as a mirror that reflects the ways in which, in our most depraved state, we can view other human beings. Pornography demonstrates to women the reality that men are prone to selfishness, domination and violence. Pornography ultimately forces men to this realization about themselves as well.

Pornography and the masturbation it fuels are sins committed against one's own body (1 Cor 6:17). Our bodies are temples of God (1 Cor 6:12-20), and whenever we engage in sexual sin alone or with another, we dishonor the image of God in all parties involved. The lack of respect for the image of God and our embodied nature damages us at every level and impairs our ability to know God and others rightly. Pornography affects those who are closest to the offenders, particularly wives and children. Both husband and wife suffer when pornographic infidelity creeps into the marriage covenant. The necessary healing can often be long and painful. In some cases, divorce can occur. There can also be professional or ministry consequences as well. The viewing of pornography and sexually acting out may not meet the letter of the law for adultery (Mt 5:28), but it certainly meets the spirit of the law. Pornography fuels our sexual drive by directing it toward objectification of the image of God in others and using them for personal consumption. The result is that we drift into isolation and depravity that we were not created for (Eph 4:19; Rom 1:24-28).

Whenever we sin we grieve the heart of God and we defile his image (Eph 4:31). Each time a man views pornography he impairs the ability of the Holy Spirit to direct him toward sanctification, and he slips further into depravity (1 Thess 5:19). The more a man views pornography, the less likely he will be inclined to seek out God and live a life of holiness. With repeated viewing and acting out, he isolates himself and becomes more likely to be given over to the desires of his twisted and depraved heart.

The more pornography a man views, the less freedom he has over what he thinks and pursues. He becomes enslaved to his sin (Rom 6:16). Because his sexuality is core to his essence, the lie of sexual fulfillment appeals to him at every level (neurological, psychological and social) and ultimately disfigures his nature. It creates moral and emotional confusion that prevents him from finding fulfillment in the manner he is created to find it. He consumes an offering of pleasure when his true need is for intimacy. He longs to be known as good and to speak goodness into the sexuality of others, yet he finds decreased ability to enjoy the full humanity of others and unable to speak to anything other than their suitability to stimulate him. The need for transcendence is met only with an increased sense of isolation and an acute awareness of his own smallness.

Sexually acting out in response to pornography creates sexual associations that are stored as hormonal and neurological habits. These associations are seared into the fabric of the brain. These memories can then be pulled up at any time and replayed as private sexual fantasies. In sexual fantasy, the neurological circuit is replayed, further strengthening it. The result is an increase in autonomic sexual arousal, which requires an outlet. These memories and fantasies keep him in bondage and worsen the consequences of the earlier behavior. It can prevent him from being truly present in a marriage, being more preoccupied with the images than focused on his wife.

Pornography corrupts the intimacy that a man and woman can experience together because of the baggage it inherently brings with it.

Men believe they should make love like a porn star to a woman who should look like a porn star. Rather than being who he is with the woman he is with, he measures his performance against the performers he has seen. (Porn stars often refer to themselves as "performers," suggesting the sexual encounter is not an emotionally real one.) He evaluates the staged intimacy between two performers (not himself and his wife) against his sexual relations with his wife. He cannot be fully present; he is assessing his "performance." Intimacy in marriage is further corrupted by the man measuring the woman he is with (whom he should be focused on) against the woman on the screen. Pornography is the recording of sexual intimacy between two human beings, whether authentic or not. When it is consumed by another, it intrudes on how that person is able to be intimate with their partner.

REFERENCES

U.S. Attorney General's commission on pornography. 1986. Available from <http://www.porn-report.com/>.

Ariely, D., and G. Loewenstein. 2006. The heat of the moment: the effect of sexual arousal on sexual decision making. *Journal of Behavioral Decision Making* 19, no. 2: 87.

Balswick, J. K., and J. O. Balswick. 1999. *Authentic human sexuality: An integrated Christian approach.* Downers Grove, IL: InterVarsity Press.

Brooks, G. R. 1995. *The centerfold syndrome.* San Francisco: Jossey-Bass.

Jensen, Robert. 2007. *Getting off: Pornography and the end of masculinity.* Cambridge, MA: South End Press.

Kelsey, M., and B. Kelsey. 1999. *Sacrament of sexuality: The spirituality and psychology of sex.* Rockport, MA: Element Inc.

Loftus, D. 2002. *Watching sex: How men really respond to pornography.* New York: Thunder's Mouth Press.

Maltz, Wendy, and Larry Maltz. 2008. *The porn trap.* New York: HarperCollins.

Paul, P. 2005. *Pornified: How pornography is transforming our lives,*

our relationships, and our families. New York: Times Books.
Schwarz, N. 2000. Emotion, cognition, and decision making. *Cognition & Emotion* 14, no. 4: 433-40.
Seymour, Ben, and Ray Dolan. 2008. Emotion, Decision Making, and the Amygdala. *Neuron* 58, no. 5 (6/12): 662-71.

3

The Consequences of Porn

"Then he said to me, 'Son of man, have you seen what the elders of the house of Israel are doing in the dark, each in his room of pictures? For they say, "The Lord does not see us, the Lord has forsaken the land."' He said also to me, 'You will see still greater abominations that they commit.'"

EZEKIEL 8:12-13

NO MATTER WHERE WE GO, GOD SEES US. He sees what we do in our secret hiding places. We may think that no one knows our most private moments, but God is there with us. As a man's relationship with pornography becomes stronger, it becomes increasingly difficult to hide. There may be a season of deception, but it will eventually come to the light. God sees and grieves the things that are done behind the walls of men's homes, dormitory rooms and offices. And sexual sin can be very ugly when it comes to light.

It's not difficult to imagine how a lack of control in one's sexual life can lead to a variety of problems; just look at the headlines. The sexual activities of celebrities and politicians are routinely exposed in the news. Sexual violence against women and children is also frequently reported. It is common to hear of community members such as school-teachers, lawyers, factory workers and pastors who are guilty of inappropriate sexual conduct or who have exposed themselves to inappropriate sexual material. The problems that result range from practical social consequences (loss of job, reputation and finances) to deeper emotional, relational and spiritual problems.

In his book *Watching Sex: How Men Really Respond to Pornography*, David Loftus shares his findings from a non-scientific survey of 150 men (Loftus, 2002). In his interviews he attempted to discover the reasons why these men regularly viewed pornography. Loftus listed five major reasons why these men view porn, and I have included some additional thoughts on them below.

> *Curiosity.* They just wanted to know the many forms that women had, or how a clothed woman looked naked (i.e., celebrities in *Playboy*). This can also be compounded when there is a moral dimension to it—the allure of the forbidden.

> *Play of fantasy.* These men long to imagine a world that is all that they want it to be; they are dissatisfied with this world and long to participate in another.

> *Pleasure of surrender.* The giving in to the pleasures of the sexual excitement and response (orgasm); the need to surrender into something greater than themselves (i.e., transcendence).

> *Importance of women's pleasure.* It is important that they see women in ecstasy; they understand the relational aspect of transcendence and wish to share it.

> *Appreciation of the female form.* They are drawn to the beauty of the female form; it becomes an altar at which they worship.

In addition to these reasons, it has been my experience that many men who have problems with pornography show a number of significant psychological patterns. Not all men have them, but often it is helpful in seeing how these factors may contribute to their problems.

1. *Controlling.* A need to manipulate their environment and others around them in order to have a sense of security.

2. *Highly introverted.* Internally focused and having little meaningful social interaction with others. They are predisposed to being isolated.

3. *Have high anxiety.* Easily stressed by family life, work or dealing with expectations placed on them by others.

4. *Narcissistic.* A need to be admired by those around them as exceptional in some way. They seek admiration, not affirmation.

5. *Curious.* Natural inquisitiveness about things, people, places, etc. (not just sexual). A strong desire for novel experiences.

6. *Have low self-esteem.* Men who feel inadequate with women or with their fellow men. They have a need for affirmation, not admiration.

7. *Depressed.* Men who have a level of emotion that is regularly low and are predisposed toward depression.

8. *Dissociative.* Men who separate or suppress their emotions and refuse to maintain an integrated, holistic view of themselves.

9. *Distractible.* Men who have difficulty keeping their attention on things; unable to control their impulse to move on to something more interesting.

Men who have these personality traits or struggle with these issues seem to be easy prey for pornography. When more than one of these factors is present, the predisposition to porn use increases.

SEXUAL INSTINCT

The simplest explanation for why men view pornography (or solicit prostitutes) is they are driven to seek out sexual intimacy. Satisfying this drive is pleasurable. Sexual intercourse and the naked form of women are enjoyable, as designed by God to be. If the goal of our sexuality is to experience pleasure, then it should come as no surprise that many men take a shortcut to sexual pleasure via pornography and masturbation.

But there are other, deeper reasons for our sexuality. If there were no limitations on sexual intercourse, then it would be logical to assume that the primary purpose of intercourse is pleasure. But there are clear biblical restrictions and limitations on sexual intercourse (Lev 18). What are these limitations on our sexuality for? What do they tell us about the primary purpose of sexual relations and why restrictions are needed? What happens when men misunderstand this drive as inherently about sexual gratification and not about relational intimacy? They treat others as commodities to be consumed for satisfaction, rather than people to be bonded with through a shared experience.

THE OLDEST PROFESSION
Estimates range from 7 to 39 percent of men worldwide solicit and have sex with prostitutes (Westerhoff, 2008, pp. 62-67). There are two major schools of thought regarding why men seek out sex with prostitutes or pornography. Some are of the opinion that pornography and prostitution serve as a balm for dealing with common psychological afflictions. A need for sexual fulfillment due to the absence of a willing partner, a craving for sexual anger, the excitement of a "romantic" encounter or a way to let off steam are all possible reasons.

Others, however, suggest that the chronic pursuit of prostitutes and pornography are the result of a need to dominate and control women. Researchers reviewing the personality profiles of johns charged with solicitation of a prostitute revealed a tendency for risk-taking and unprotected sex. Men who had more aggressive personalities demanded sex without condoms. Another study indicated that these johns were sexually frustrated or were hedonists interested in living out their fantasies. Some men go to prostitutes to experiment sexually in ways that their wives or girlfriends may not be willing to. This desire for sexual creativity as part of a financial transaction offers the promise of increased sexual fulfillment.

But some researchers have suggested that johns believe that they are involved in a genuine intimate relationship with the prostitute. The emotional and psychological needs met cause them to become regulars. Nearly two thirds of the johns were repeat customers (one in four having over 100 encounters with the same prostitute). After finding a "safe" sexual partner, they return again and again. Because of this need for intimacy, many johns will discuss the personalities of their regular prostitute. The emotional exchange that occurs for these men, who long for intimacy, is powerful and real. The relationship becomes a pseudo-marriage; sex without the messiness of commitment. In the absence of a socially approved or morally sanctioned relationship with a woman, some men gravitate to prostitution. It is not uncommon for johns to seek to extend the social nature of the encounter, making it more than just about intercourse. They offer personal information about themselves (justifying or rationalizing their solicitation) and also ask about the prostitute's life.

What makes pornography different from prostitution is that there is no personal exchange between the image and the viewer. The absence of any real relationship makes the pornography that much more hollow after failing to deliver on its promise of intimacy. Not surprisingly, men who are looking for intimacy will often progress to more advanced cybersexual encounters. Webcams, chat rooms and services like Adult Friend Finder offer opportunities to connect with real people. These may be mediated over the Internet or may lead to real-world encounters.

So why do men turn to prostitutes or pornography rather than a wife? Again, the reason may appear obvious. Women are complicated and usually expect a level of commitment in exchange for sexual favors. By using pornography or a prostitute, he avoids most of the work that goes into a relationship with a real woman. There are no worries about rejected advances, headaches, moodiness or carryover from arguments earlier in the day. Pornography and prostitutes are on-demand outlets for sexual needs, and if any unmet emotional need gets taken care of, it is icing on the cake.

POWER PLAY

It is possible that pornography and soliciting prostitutes are avenues by which men exercise a need to be in control. Because women have the psychological power of withholding their sexuality, men prey on women's financial need and use money to overcome this barrier. Pornography and sex with a prostitute become means by which a man can feel that he is in control or effective, or in the case of misogyny, can get revenge. This feeling of being in control is also what many rapists refer to when asked why they force themselves on their victims. It becomes less about sexual gratification and more about the control they have over their victims. It is not about intimacy; it is about power.

While some men may think of their relationship with a prostitute or their webcam sexual partner as a person they are connecting with, others think of the women as product to be consumed. The idea of an intimate relationship is distasteful to them. The presence of misogynistic pornography available on the web that demeans women is expansive. Indeed the use of the term "material" when describing the pornography reveals the depths of such consumer-oriented objectification. By being coerced, forced or psychologically trapped into selling their bodies, women's emotions are splintered from their bodies. Both are fractured in this exchange; the emotional, psychological, physiological and spiritual dimensions of themselves are disintegrated.

Human beings are not a commodity. When forced to act as one, the emotional and psychological damage is severe. Many women in porn and prostitution have been sexually, physically, emotionally and verbally abused by men. Abuse at the hands of fathers, family members, boyfriends and others fracture what was meant to be whole. In spite of what those in the sex industry might say, prostitution and pornography are not industries that psychologically healthy women seek out. Financial difficulties, substance abuse and psychological brokenness are the reasons most women enter into pornography and the sex trade.

COGNITIVE CONSEQUENCES

Viewing pornography is not an emotionally or physiologically neutral experience. It is fundamentally different from looking at black and white photos of the Lincoln Memorial or taking in a color map of the provinces of Canada. Men are reflexively drawn to the content of pornographic material. As such, pornography has wide-reaching effects to energize a man toward intimacy. It is not a neutral stimulus. It draws us in. Porn is vicarious and voyeuristic at its core, but it is also something more. Porn is a whispered promise. It promises more sex, better sex, endless sex, sex on demand, more intense orgasms, experiences of transcendence. Time spent with porn prevents the user from engaging in real relationships with real people who can better meet their needs.

Although many men claim that they are in control, the reality is that their behavioral patterns show a lack of control. They are in denial, not control. So what happens when confronted with this reality? They claim that they do not want to stop, deny, minimize, normalize, justify, rationalize or celebrate their relationship with porn. It becomes an insidious cycle that often ends in shame.

In his book *Out of the Shadows*, Dr. Patrick Carnes describes sex addiction as "a pathological relationship with a mood-altering experience" (Carnes, 2001). It acts as polydrug, delivering emotional and sensory excitation and energizing a man sexually. This mood-altering experience is rooted in the ability that sexual acting out has on changing the emotional state of the person involved in it (Ariely and Loewenstein, 2006, p. 87). The emphasis, though, on the mood-altering effects of viewing pornography and sexually acting out provides only a narrow snapshot into the mind of the male struggling with pornography. There are multiple reasons why someone seeks out a mood-altering experience: boredom, frustration, anxiety. Salience refers to pornography's ability to dominate the person's life and behaviors. They become increasingly preoccupied with acquiring, viewing and acting out to the point that it consumes their thought life. Spending time on sexual pursuits becomes the norm, not the exception for their daily activities. As they become more bound to and consumed by the pornography, these "rushes" can be felt even as they begin the ritual preparation for the next time they act out.

COGNITIVE TRAPS

Aside from the issues surrounding how men think about their viewing of pornography already mentioned, men fall into other cognitive traps when dealing with those who confront them about it (Reid and Gray, 2006).

1. *Entitlement: "I've earned this."* Some men feel that their lot in life requires that they receive some sort of special treatment. They may feel that they have been given the short end of the stick by God, their parents, the culture, their children or their church. They may feel that they should be given special permission to have this one outlet as their reward for their suffering. Others may feel that they may be better than everyone else and should be given more privileges in this area. Because of their unique and special position, they are exempted from being held to the same moral standards. Entitlement is a significant problem with men who have a narcissistic need for affirmation at the core of their problems.

2. *Omniscience: "I know what you are thinking."* A man may feel that he knows the intentions or responses of others, and he questions the motives of those who are trying to help him. He may think that his wife is just trying to restrict his freedom, his pastor is being holier-than-thou, or his therapist is just seeing him for the money. By assuming that he knows the motives of others trying to help him, he absolves himself of his inappropriate behavior.

3. *Altruism: "I am keeping it quiet to protect others."* Someone who has a problem with pornography may continue to conceal his problem because he thinks it is best for those he loves to be unaware of his involvement. He believes that it would be too painful for his wife to discover his problem, or that his children would be ostracized if others found out. By hiding his problem he is a noble protector of those he loves. Underneath this error in thinking is the reality that he would be pained by the pain of those he loves. As a result, he avoids disclosing his involvement and justifies it as an altruistic act.

4. *Deception: "Nope, not me."* Whether through direct lies of commission (stating falsehoods), omission (only telling part of the truth) or

assent (remaining silent and allowing the silence to be interpreted as innocence), deception is a skill that many men have honed as part of their descent into depravity. Unfortunately, this skill is so well practiced on others that a man may effectively deceive himself with respect to his motives, frequency of use and the depth to which his pornography problem has developed. He may not be in denial, but he is so deceived that he really does not see his world falling apart around him.

5. *Blaming/Victimization: "It's her fault."* When a man refuses to accept responsibility for his behaviors, he will find a scapegoat. It may be a wife who doesn't want to be sexually intimate as frequently as he does, stress at work, unreasonable expectations placed on him by God or the irresistible sensuality of the models. By playing the victim, the user attempts to absolve himself of his guilt.

6. *Pride: "I am right, you are wrong."* It might be that a man's identity is so wrapped up in being right and his sense of superiority that any admission of wrong behavior is not possible. A prideful person refuses to be humble and acknowledge his problem. His inability to admit his sin prevents him from starting on the path to becoming healthy, whole and sanctified.

7. *Objectification: "They're just models."* Part of the problem with pornography is that it causes men to look at women as sexual parts rather than human beings. The objectification of women reduces them to objects for sexual stimulation and is demeaning.

8. *Distraction: "I've been really stressed lately."* By shifting the focus away from the inappropriate behavior to something else, like difficulty at work, a man can become too focused on what he believes is a justified cause. He redirects attention toward (but may not blame) some other issue as more important. The stress at work is a more significant problem to deal with, not his pornography compulsion.

9. *Revenge: "This'll show her/him."* Some men will purposely view pornography as a way of wounding someone. A husband can sexually act out as a way of expressing anger against his wife. An employee will act out at work to get back at a boss who has given him a bad yearly evaluation. This twisted form of thinking sees the problem behavior

as a way of wounding someone without their knowledge. In a marriage it can be used to inflict the wounds of emotional adultery without catching an STD. In a dating relationship it can be a way of releasing aggression about a girlfriend's insistence on keeping her virginity. Regardless of the situation, viewing porn and sexually acting out become acts of aggression in the heart of the user. Pornography provokes and has at its core an element of anger, not joy or love. Men are invited into love and joy, but pornography provokes to anger, frustration, hostility and distrust. These emotions underlie the connection between pornography and sexual aggression toward women and can be seen when it is used for revenge.

These are only a sampling of some of the effects that repeated exposure to pornography can have on a man's mind. They are not exclusive to men, as women who struggle with intimacy issues and consume porn regularly may also think in these ways, but they appeal to many of the psychological Achilles' heels that a man may have.

There are many psychological, social, professional and spiritual side effects of regular pornography use. They may include increased callousness toward women, decreased satisfaction with sexual relationships, diminished attitude of love toward existing partners, dissatisfaction with one's own body, an inability to control sexual arousal, shame about one's own sexuality, feeling separated from God, an increase in deviant sexual fantasies, irritability, a preoccupation with acquiring additional sexually explicit material, increased interpersonal conflict, paranoia about being caught as well as lack of inhibition in other aspects of their life, such as alcohol and drug use or gambling.

Many other internal and external factors are believed to be involved in pornography viewing. Inconsistent parental nurturing and love, parental betrayal or abandonment (real or perceived) are significant factors that can lead to emotional issues driving the sexual need for attachment. Insufficient parental teaching and modeling may lead to confusion about how to respond appropriately to sexual arousal. Child abuse, early sexualization and stress are also contributing external factors. Internal factors such as emotional insensitivity and a controlling nature can also contribute to the problem.

Pornography offers an answer to how a man should meet his body's demands. It gives him control and appeals to a sense that we should be responsible for satisfying our own needs. It provides an amount of predictability; we have confidence that it is available when we need it. It provides a "safe" way of reducing sexual tension. It can also be used to provide relief from relational pain with others. It offers a way to deal with loneliness and shame. Porn is a transient way to find a sense of fulfillment, avoid pain or get through the day. Unfortunately pornography usually just makes things worse.

The degree to which men develop problems with pornography is an indication of the intensity of their unmet internal needs and desires. As these needs become more intense, the sights and stimulation of porn and an accompanying orgasm become more fleeting as tolerance develops. Increased tolerance means that progression from softcore nakedness to more explicit hardcore materials is necessary to produce arousal. The continued unmet need for emotional intimacy or unresolved stress makes matters worse. Feelings of shame and anxiety produced by the fear of being caught increase as well.

RETHINKING TYPOLOGY

Men who struggle with pornography and masturbation commonly refer to it as an addiction. The term "addiction" has typically been reserved for maladaptive behavioral patterns surrounding drugs. For most addictive drugs, their effect on the brain makes them addictive. With substance addictions, the drug is somehow taken into the body. Typical intake routes include oral ingestion, intravenous insertion or inhalation. The drug is then distributed throughout the body where it is metabolized and discarded. If it is a substance that acts on the brain and nervous system, it may produce a psychoactive event. If it dulls pain (aspirin), speeds up thought (caffeine) or alters mood (antidepressants), we may have little problem with the ingestion of such a drug. But what makes drugs of abuse and addiction problematic is that they act on regions and circuits in the brain that underlie pleasure, reinforcement and our ability to discern what external cues are important for our well-being.

So what if we find that pornography works through the same neural circuit, has the same effects with respect to tolerance and withdrawal, and has every other hallmark of an addiction? It is important to notice that the DSM-IV (the *Diagnostic and Statistical Manual of the American Psychiatric Association*) criteria for addictions are primarily based in the behavioral and cognitive realm and less on the physiological. We consider gambling an addiction, so why should we not grant the same status of addiction to pornography viewing, especially in light of the clinical evidence?

While the terms "sexual addiction" and "pornography addiction" are currently being debated in the psychological and medical communities, there is still a great deal that we do not know about how pornography affects individuals. When I was young my dad told me, "If it looks like a duck, walks like a duck and quacks like a duck, it's a duck." So does pornography look, walk and quack like addictive drugs? Is pornography an addiction? Or is there a better way to talk about the problems that men have with pornography? I think a better use of terminology can not only be helpful in the diagnosis and treatment of pornography problems, but also help reduce some of the unhealthy shame often associated with it.

Ask someone what an addiction is and chances are you will hear a variety of answers. Some people will give you descriptions of people in bondage to a behavior or object. The drug addict in the back alley shooting up, or the alcoholic passed out in their living room with an empty bottle may come to people's minds. Others may describe people who are addicted to video games or even relationships. Still others will describe someone stuck on something that they need in order to function. In fact, some proudly proclaim their addiction to everything from coffee, soda, cigars, gambling, Guitar Hero or Halo 3 all the way to pornography.

All drugs have several effects on the body when we ingest them. What is called the *main effect* is usually determined by the purpose of administering the drug. It is the reason that we take the drug or medication in the first place. It stops us from coughing, makes the headache go away, eases the pain or speeds up the healing process. But drugs don't care about why you are taking them. For the most part, they are not "target" specific. They are distributed throughout the body and affect the body's organs in different ways. This is why most drugs have *side effects*. These side effects are the result of the drug acting in places other than where you need it. For example, if you have high blood pressure you may take a medication that reduces your blood pressure. But that drug may also have the side effects of dry mouth, drowsiness or nausea.

Use of a drug differs from *misuse* of a drug. A person may misuse a drug by taking it for an effect it doesn't produce. A person may misuse aspirin by taking it to gain better eyesight. Misuse is the use of a substance for which it is not an effective treatment. It doesn't work, but any harm from its use is minimal. Misuse is different from *abuse*. Drug abuse is best described as taking a drug or medication to solve a problem for which it is not well suited and in a way harmful to the person. A person who abuses alcohol drinks to deal with stress, anxiety or perhaps depression and masks these by the effects of the alcohol. It is one thing to have a single glass of wine with dinner to heighten the taste of the food you are eating. It is another to drink an entire bottle of wine so that you do not have to deal with the stress of your marriage. With abuse, a substance is used for a purpose that is better addressed by some other means. A person can use alcohol without abusing it.

Not all use constitutes abuse, nor is all abuse *dependency*. Dependency can be seen along two dimensions. *Physical dependency* is the process by which the body comes to rely on the presence of the substance in order for it to function normally. *Psychological dependency* is the result of repeated use of a substance where the person believes that they need to have it in order to function. Often people confuse physical and psychological dependency. For example, marijuana does not elicit physiological dependency. However, people can become psychologically dependent on it. Dependency is also different from tolerance. *Tolerance* is when, as a result of exposure to the substance, the body adjusts so that later exposure to the same levels of the substance results in a lesser effect. If I take the same dose of a drug over and over and my body begins to tolerate it, I will need to take a higher dose of the drug in order for it to have the same effect that it did with a lower dose the first time.

Many people make the assumption that abuse, physiological dependency, psychological dependency and tolerance are synonymous with addiction. Once again, this is not the case. The use of the word "addiction" carries with it a substantial amount of cultural, medical and therapeutic baggage. The label of "addict" may lead to particular beliefs about the nature of the person (i.e., a person with significant character or personality issues), the manner in which they should be helped (i.e., psychotherapy, inpatient care) and the level to which the person should be held legally and/or morally accountable for their actions (i.e., does the addict really have the capacity to make the right choices, to choose not to steal to support their habit, if the addiction is so severe?).

In many ways, the notion of the "addict" has been shaped by hundreds of years of social and religious perspectives on people that have become chemically addicted to substances. Some chemical addictions are socially acceptable or tolerated (caffeine, alcohol). The hallmarks of an *addiction* are that there are a number of clear behavioral criteria, cognitive patterns and neurological systems that underlie the addictive pattern.

PORN ADDICTION

"Pornography addiction" is a phrase that some clinicians are resistant to and others have embraced. While it is not currently a part of the DSM-IV, I will use the term loosely for now because of the similarities that are found when looking at the criteria for substance addiction (American Psychiatric Association, 2000). When considering whether pornography can be addictive, it is helpful to go to the DSM-IV for guidance. It is the tool that psychiatrists and psychotherapists use to diagnose problems of addiction. I have modified the DSM-IV criteria for "substance abuse" and "substance dependency" to present a picture of what "pornography addiction" might look like from a clinician's perspective.

DSM-IV SUBSTANCE ABUSE CRITERIA [SUBSTITUTING TERMINOLOGY FOR PORNOGRAPHY USE]

1. Recurrent [viewing pornographic material or images with or without sexual acting out] resulting in a failure to fulfill major role obligations at work, school, or home (such as repeated absences or poor work performance, absences, suspensions, or expulsions from school; or neglect of children or household)

2. Recurrent [viewing pornographic material or images with or without sexual acting out] in situations in which it is physically hazardous

3. Recurrent [viewing pornographic material or images with or without sexual acting out]-related legal problems (such as arrests for [viewing pornographic material or images with or without sexual acting out]-related disorderly conduct)

4. Continued [viewing pornographic material or images with or without sexual acting out] despite having persistent or recurrent social or interpersonal problems caused or exacerbated by their effects (for example, arguments with spouse about consequences)

DSM-IV SUBSTANCE DEPENDENCY CRITERIA [SUBSTITUTING TERMINOLOGY FOR PORNOGRAPHY USE]

Tentatively defined as a maladaptive pattern of [viewing pornographic material or images with or without sexual acting out] leading to clinically significant impairment or distress, as manifested by three (or more) of the following, occurring any time in the same 12-month period:

1. Tolerance, as defined by either of the following:

    (a) A need for markedly increased amounts of the [viewing pornographic material or images with or without sexual acting out] to achieve intoxication or the desired effect, or:

    (b) Markedly diminished effect of sexual satisfaction when engaging in [viewing pornographic material or images with or without sexual acting out].

2. Withdrawal, as manifested by either of the following:

    (a) The characteristic withdrawal syndrome for the [viewing pornographic material or images with or without sexual acting out], or:

    (b) The same (or closely related) [viewing pornographic material or images with or without sexual acting out] is taken to relieve or avoid withdrawal symptoms.

3. The [viewing pornographic material or images with or without sexual acting out] is often progressive (needed in larger amounts or over a longer period than intended).

4. There is a persistent desire or unsuccessful efforts to cut down or control [viewing pornographic material or images with or without sexual acting out] use.

5. A great deal of time is spent in activities necessary to obtain the [viewing pornographic material or images with or without sexual acting out], use the [viewing pornographic material or images with or without sexual acting out], or recover from their effects.

6. Important social, occupational, or recreational activities are given up or reduced because of [viewing pornographic material or images with or without sexual acting out].

7. The [viewing pornographic material or images with or without sexual acting out] are continued despite knowledge of having a persistent physical or psychological problem that is likely to have been caused or exacerbated

by the [viewing pornographic material or images with or without sexual acting out].

Notice the emphasis on abuse and dependency, tolerance and withdrawal. Addiction is characterized by compulsion, loss of control and continued use in spite of adverse consequences (Holden, 2001, pp. 980-82). The compulsive behavior is reinforcing (rewarding or pleasurable) initially, but tolerance and dependency lead to its decreasing effectiveness to produce the pleasure. Eventually the individual loses the ability to limit intake and the addiction process progresses. The ability of the drug to produce the associated pleasure is replaced by a need to fend off withdrawal. But this pattern does not always fit many who struggle with pornography.

PORN COMPULSIVITY AND IMPULSIVENESS

Some men do not have pornography addictions characterized by escalating, damaging and risky behaviors in the pursuit of a high. Perhaps they use pornography as a way of dealing with the sexual tension resulting from their obsessive sexual fantasies. Or perhaps they view pornography and act out as a way of dealing with stress in their lives. A *compulsion* is a behavior that a person engages in as a way of dealing with excessive anxiety or fear. Often associated with obsessions and diagnosed as obsessive-compulsive disorder (OCD), compulsions are ritualistic behaviors engaged in as the result of obsessing or thinking about something to the point of creating psychological and physical anxiety that needs to be resolved.

The majority of people use the Internet without major problems of compulsive online use. Unfortunately, however, approximately 1 percent of online users can spend over forty hours a week online in sexually related activities such as viewing pornography, searching for pornography and chatting in sex-oriented chat rooms. This group of individuals, mostly men, can have significant problems in a variety of areas of their lives, from workplace to home (Cooper et al., 1999, pp.

154-64). While many psychologists, medical practitioners and theorists have a variety of very valid views on how to describe these individuals, there is little doubt that something is going on with this group. What exactly is going on here, and how should we name it?

Some indicators that an individual is struggling with a compulsive online problem include:

1. Excessive personal (non-work related) use of more than 20 hours a week

2. Neglect or avoidance of previously rewarding personal relationships or interaction with peers

3. Depression (either short- or long-term)

4. Pursuit of "highs" that have been experienced while online

5. A false perception of intimacy or pseudo-intimacy

6. Internet becomes the source of resolving sexual difficulties, releasing sexual frustration or unfocused sexual energy

7. A history of sexual problems

What seems to be important in determining whether or not a behavior is considered to be compulsive or addictive is that it meets three criteria:

1. There is an inability to choose whether or not to do the behavior (compulsivity).

2. The behavior continues in spite of negative consequences that the individual is plainly aware of.

3. Thoughts centering on the behavior (i.e., when is the next time it can be done, how to acquire the necessary items to do it, etc.) take up a significant amount of the person's cognitive life (obsession).

Another possibility is that a man may just have difficulty controlling his sexual response to arousing stimuli. He may not go through his day fantasizing or obsessing about women, but when the thought strikes him, he acts on it. This man does not have a compulsive problem, but a problem with *impulse control*. Other impulse disorders, such as attention deficit disorder (ADD), have at their root an inability to inhibit acting out in response to sudden urges or emotions. In this instance, a man may have problems with more than porn. He may gamble, spend excessively and spontaneously engage in risky behavior.

Those with impulse control problems do not consider the consequences of their actions. It is not that they are immune to the consequences. They simply act before they think. Addiction professionals who encounter both compulsive and impulsive sexual acting-out behaviors in their patients have experienced paradigm and nomenclature communication difficulties with mental health professionals and managed care organizations that use DSM terminology and diagnostic criteria. This difficulty in communication has fueled skepticism among some psychiatrists and other mental health professionals regarding the case for including sexual addiction as a mental disorder.

As a pattern of out-of-control behavior continues, there are significant and severe consequences. The user is unable to stop his use despite repeated attempts to limit or reduce their porn usage. It can escalate into high-risk behaviors (viewing materials in public), and the amount of time and resources devoted to pornography increases in spite of a perception of only a short time passing. They have significant changes in mood and often neglect social, professional, recreational and physical (i.e., eating, sleeping) opportunities and needs. Much of the time is spent on the Internet seeking opportunities for sexual arousal or cybersexual exchanges.

Rather than paint all men with the same brush and focus on the high of sexual release alone, it may be more beneficial to spend more time figuring out what the core of the problem is. Rather than a need to chase down the orgasmic high, running after a pot of gold at the end of the rainbow, many men are unable to control their thoughts (compulsivity), fail to inhibit their sexual arousal (impulsivity), soothe their feelings of inadequacy (depression) or use pornography as a stress reducer. You wouldn't treat a depressed person like you would a narcissist, and you wouldn't medicate someone with attention deficit disorder like you would someone with low self-esteem. The parts of the brain that are involved of each of these problems are different, so shouldn't the way we understand how to treat these problems mirror that? As men gain a greater understanding of why they struggle with porn, the emphasis on redeeming and rewiring themselves neurologically should be informed by these embodied facts.

REFERENCES

American Psychiatric Association. 2000. *Diagnostic and statistical manual of mental disorders,* 4th ed., text revision (DSM-IV-TR). Washington, DC: American Psychiatric Association.

Ariely, D., and G. Loewenstein. 2006. The heat of the moment: The effect of sexual arousal on sexual decision making. *Journal of Behavioral Decision Making* 19, no. 2: 87.

Carnes, P. 2001. *Out of the shadows: Understanding sexual addiction.* Center City, MN: Hazelden Publishing & Educational Services.

Cooper, A., C. R. Scherer, S. C. Boies and B. L. Gordon. 1999. Sexuality on the Internet: From sexual exploration to pathological expression. *Professional psychology, research and practice* 30, no. 2: 154-64.

Holden, C. 2001. "Behavioral" addictions: Do they exist? *Science* 294, no. 5544: 980-82.

Loftus, D. 2002. *Watching sex: How men really respond to pornography.* New York: Thunder's Mouth Press.

Reid, R. C., and D. Gray. 2006. *Confronting your spouse's pornography problem.* Sandy, UT: Silverleaf Press.

Westerhoff, N. 2008. Why Do Men Buy Sex? *Scientific American Mind* 62.

4

Your Brain on Porn

IF YOU'VE EVER ENTERED A MAJOR ELECTRONICS store that carries high definition (HD) televisions, you've probably seen the difference between standard and HD images. There is usually an HD television with a split screen showing the differences between the old-fashioned, standard television version and the newer, life-like HD images. The standard television system seems dull and uninteresting when contrasted to the same set of images shown on an HD system. The radiance and fine details of an HD system can be breathtaking. But having an HD television is not enough to get this glorious visual experience. You can't take a standard image and make it HD. An HD signal from your programming provider, an HD receiver and an HD display (television or monitor) all have to be connected to each other in order to get this effect. All three elements must be in place—signal, receiver and monitor—in order to experience HD in its fullness.

Pornography has a similar effect on men due to the uniqueness of our ability to pick up the signal, receive it and experience it. Pornographic images are inherently different from other signals. Images of nudity or sexual intercourse are distinct, different from what we experience as part of our everyday visual experience. They are analogous to the HD signal. The male brain is the built like an ideal pornography receiver, wired to be on the alert for these images of nakedness. The male brain and our conscious visual experience is the internal monitor where we perceive them. The images of sexuality grab our attention, jumping out and hypnotizing a man like an HD television among a sea of standard televisions.

THE VISUAL MAGNETISM OF PORNOGRAPHY

Human sexuality affects every aspect of human life, but sexual acts are generally understood as private acts, taking place in the bedroom. We live in a culture that is clothed, and we do not regularly stumble across people having sex in public. We have laws against nudity and performing sexual acts in public. This cultural reality along with the intuitive notion that sex is a private, intimate act makes pornography so qualitatively different from the majority of our everyday visual experience. Our culture has trained us so that there is something about the naked form that is distinctive. When we come across it, we reflexively turn our attention toward it. But why do so many men find it difficult to look away after that first glance? Perhaps it is because their receiver is merely locking onto this strong signal.

A man's brain is a sexual mosaic influenced by hormone levels in the womb and in puberty and molded by his psychological experience. Male brains can be very different from female brains because of this (Arnold, 2004, pp. 701-8; Ariely and Loewenstein. 2006, p. 87; Baron-Cohen, Lutchmaya and Knickmeyer, 2004; Brizendine, 2006; Cahill, 2006, p. 477). Although neither superior nor inferior, they are very different in the way they detect stimuli, process information and respond to emotions. This is important because men detect sexual cues rapidly when it comes to nakedness or sex-related stimuli. Men seem to be more sensitive to visual cues for sexual arousal (Lykins, Meana and Kambe, 2006, pp. 569-75; Janssen, Carpenter and Graham, 2003, pp. 243-51; Karama et al., 2002, p. 1; Koukounas and McCabe, 1997, pp. 221-30). The visual scanning of the naked image has a power to it that forces itself onto the male brain. The peculiar proficiency that the male brain has to relay this signal, combined with a man's personal history and thought habits (his experience with looking at pornography), are why so many men have difficulty looking away. The signal is received and then projected onto the display, the visual experience of the viewer. The depiction of nudity and sexual acts have a hypnotic effect and the ability to hold their attention similar to an HD television.

As men fall deeper into the mental habit of fixating on these images, the exposure to them creates neural pathways. Like a path is created in the woods with each successive hiker, so do the neural paths set the course for the next time an erotic image is viewed. Over time these neural paths become wider as they are repeatedly traveled with each exposure to pornography. They become the automatic pathway through which interactions with women are routed. The neural circuitry anchors this process solidly in the brain. With each lingering stare, pornography deepens a Grand Canyon–like gorge in the brain through which images of women are destined to flow. This extends to women that they have not seen naked or engaging in sexual acts as well. All women become potential porn stars in the minds of these men. They have unknowingly created a neurological circuit that imprisons their ability to see women rightly as created in God's image.

Repeated exposure to pornography creates a one-way neurological superhighway where a man's mental life is over-sexualized and narrowed. It is hemmed in on either side by high containment walls making escape nearly impossible. This neurological superhighway has many on-ramps. The mental life is fixated on sex, but it is intended for intimacy. It is wide—able to accommodate multiple partners, images and sexual possibilities, but it is intended to be narrow—a place for God's exclusive love to be imaged. This neurological superhighway has been reconstructed and built for speed, able to rapidly get to the climax of sexual stimulation. It is intended, however, for the slow discovery and appreciation of a loving partner. The pornography-built pathway has only a few off-ramps, leading to sexual encounters that have only a fleeting impact and hasten the need for more. But these encounters are intended to be long lasting and satisfying for both partners and have many off ramps for creative expressions of intimacy that are not genitally oriented.

BRAIN SCANNING

You may have heard on the evening news or read in a popular magazine that scientists have found the "pleasure centers" of the brain. Journalists or newscasters need only refer to dopamine or serotonin and they have instant scientific credibility. Throw in a reference to the brain or genetics and you have a rhetorical slam dunk regardless of what the topic is. This appeal to science as the most authoritative voice on any topic extends into various topics of cultural importance such as healthcare and mental health (i.e., obesity and depression), criminal behavior (i.e., brain damage and aggression), and many political hot-button issues (i.e., homosexuality, stem cell research and abortion).

In a recent study conducted at UCLA, students were asked to read an article and evaluate its credibility (McCabe and Castel, 2008, pp. 343-52). The articles were actually fictional and quite flawed with headlines such as "Playing Video Games Benefits Attention" and "Watching TV Is Related to Math Ability." The researchers found that when the article was accompanied by brain images such as those taken during functional magnetic resonance imaging or positron emission tomography, the students tended to assign greater validity to the claims of the article. Articles with brain images came across as more convincing than articles without images or with standard bar graphs and charts.

Underneath our penchant for being seduced by brain science is a sense that what is going on inside our brain is fundamental to our psychological experience. For some this knowledge is a relief. Understanding depression, an anxiety disorder, obesity or addiction as something that is a part of how they are biologically put together can be extraordinarily helpful. It may explain the difficulty they have experienced in dealing with their emotions or breaking destructive habits. For others that same knowledge might lead to a fatalist view of themselves.

Because the human brain, the source of our mental life, is such a remarkable organ, it is important to have a good understanding of how it operates. Knowledge about how it is put together and the regions having greater responsibility for the varied aspects of our psychological experience help us understand why pornography affects us the way it does. When we understand how the brain is flexible and plastic and also how it is unyielding and rigid, we can see not only how pornography can lead a person to a place of mental depravity, but also how hope for redemption and sanctification can be achieved.

THE BRAIN: MORE SIMPLE THAN YOU THINK

The human brain is an incredibly complex organ, and many people do not even bother to try to understand it. This is one of the biggest obstacles I face as a teacher with my students. But the brain is much easier to grasp than most people think. What I have found to be helpful is to focus not on the astronomical number of connections and cells, but on the organizing principles of its structure and connectivity. Focus not on its complexity, but on its major structures and functions. Once this is addressed, the rest falls into place.

The brain has three major sections that are based on what we know about how it develops. As the embryo grows, it develops what is called the neural tube. This tube is much like a garden hose capped at both ends and will form the spinal cord and the brain. As the embryo continues to grow, toward its head the neural tube develops three bumps, which eventually become the brain. These bumps are called the *hindbrain, midbrain* and *forebrain* (see table 4.1). As these regions grow they further divide into a number of regions. These subdivisions become more specialized in their function and connectivity.

HINDBRAIN: MEDULLA, PONS AND CEREBELLUM

The part of the brain closest to the spinal cord is where the hindbrain is located. The hindbrain, whose primary job is to keep us alive and to coordinate movement, has three subdivisions. At the base of the brain where it meets the spinal cord is the deepest part of the hindbrain, the *medulla* (see figure 4.2 on p. 91). The medulla is responsible for maintaining the body's vital functions such as breathing and pumping blood. Just above the medulla is the *pons*, which helps coordinate vol-

Table 4.1. Major Brain Regions

Brain Region	Primary Subdivision	Second Order Subdivision	Third Order Subdivision	Function
FOREBRAIN	Telencephalon	Cortex	Four Lobes / Multiple Gyri	1. Higher order thought processes 2. Perception
		Basal Ganglia	Striatum	1. Movement 2. Implicit learning
		Limbic System	Amygdala	Emotion
			Hippocampus	Memory
			Corpus Callosum	Connects the two hemispheres
	Diencephalon	Thalamus	1. Multiple sensory subregions 2. Lateral Geniculate Nucleus (vision)	Sensory processing
		Hypothalamus	Multiple subregions for drives	1. Primary drives (eating, drinking, sex) 2. Motivation 3. Hormonal control
MIDBRAIN	Tectum	Superior Colliculi	-	Visual reflexes
		Inferior Colliculi	-	Auditory reflexes
	Tegmentum	(Multiple subregions)	VTA	1. Arousal 2. Salience
HINDBRAIN	Pons	-	-	Movement
	Cerebellum	-	-	Movement
	Medulla	-	-	Vital life systems

untary movement. Buckled behind and interconnected with the pons is the *cerebellum*. The cerebellum has many folds and sits like a little brain tucked underneath the back end of the brain. As part of the hindbrain, the cerebellum coordinates involuntary movement, balance and posture. More recent research has suggested that the cerebellum is more than just a motor specific region; it also appears to have some involvement in emotions.

These three regions make up the deepest part of the brain, the hindbrain. Because of the importance of what they do, they are locked into their functions and connections. These brain regions have limited flexibility, and that is a good thing. Damage or dysfunction within these regions can result in severe impairment or death.

MIDBRAIN: TECTUM AND TEGMENTUM

Moving upward from the hindbrain we enter into the second developmental brain region: the *midbrain*. The midbrain and hindbrain together form the brainstem. The midbrain is subdivided into two parts whose subspecialties are critical for sensory-motor integration, neurotransmitter production and body movement. The roof of the midbrain, known as the *tectum*, has two sets of bumps that are the sensory-motor integration centers. These bumps are known as the *superior* and *inferior colliculi*. The superior colliculi process visual information and coordinate head and neck movement. Auditory information (as when reflexively craning your head to pick up where a noise is coming from) is processed by the inferior colliculi.

The floor of the midbrain is known as the tegmentum. The tegmentum has several subregions that influence consciousness, attention, sleep, wakefulness, general arousal and motor behavior. Here is where we find the first major player in what is sometimes called the "reward" system—the ventral tegmental area (VTA). The VTA manufactures the neurotransmitter dopamine and ships it up to several higher brain regions. When the VTA is activated, it releases the dopamine in these higher brain regions and acts as the neurochemical signal that something important is going on that needs significant focus (Biderman and Vessel, 2006). This dopamine release happens in anticipation of meeting drives (like eating, drinking and sex), in response to pain, and has been thought to underlie the feelings of pleasure (Hakyemez et al., 2008, pp. 2058-65; Utter and Basso, 2008, pp. 333-42; Volkow et al., 2003; Kakade and Dayan, 2002, pp. 549-59; Melis and Argiolas, 1995, pp. 19-38; van Furth, Wolterink and van Ree, 1995, pp. 162-84; Bowling, Rowlett and Bardo, 1993, pp. 885-93; Bitran and Hull, 1987). The VTA releases dopamine in response to nearly all drugs of addiction, and many disorders affecting motivation and attention such as attention deficit disorder, obsessive-compulsive disorder and behavioral addictions (i.e., sex addictions, gambling addictions, compulsive shopping) (Dalley et al., 2008; Biederman and Faraone, 2006, pp. 237-48; Andersen and Teicher, 2000, pp. 137-41, Krause et al., 2003, pp. 605-13; Krain and Castellanos, 2006, pp. 433-44; Castellanos, Glaser and Gerhardt, 2006, pp. 1-4; Sikström and Söderlund, 2007, pp. 1047-75; Russell, 2007, pp. 185-98; Ströhle et al., 2008, pp. 966-72). Dopamine release acts as a signal that teaches what is important in the environment, helps remember what the appropriate response is, and fuels the tension and craving for meeting a need (Berridge, 2007, pp. 391-431; Berridge and Winkielman, 2003, pp. 181-211).

The midbrain is similar to the hindbrain in that its connections are relatively inflexible. Damage to the midbrain is not always as debilitating when compared to the hindbrain, but dysfunction can lead to problems with sensory processing, movement, consciousness and arousal.

FOREBRAIN: DIENCEPHALON AND TELENCEPHALON
Seated above the midbrain sits the highest of the three developmental regions, the *forebrain*. The forebrain is the most complex of the three and has accordingly more subregions with more sophisticated capacities. Like the hindbrain and midbrain, the forebrain has two major subdivisions, the *diencephalon* and the *telencephalon*, but these subdivisions have subdivisions.

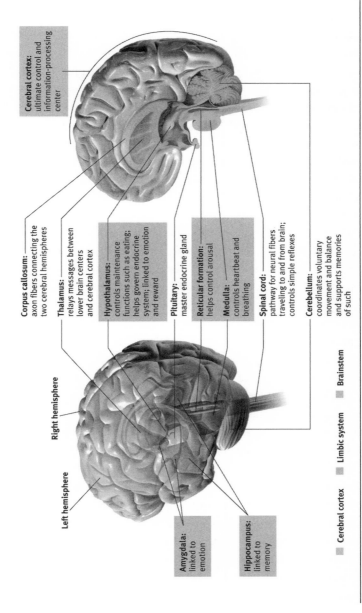

Cerebral cortex: ultimate control and information-processing center

Corpus callosum: axon fibers connecting the two cerebral hemispheres

Thalamus: relays messages between lower brain centers and cerebral cortex

Hypothalamus: controls maintenance functions such as eating; helps govern endocrine system; linked to emotion and reward

Pituitary: master endocrine gland

Reticular formation: helps control arousal

Medulla: controls heartbeat and breathing

Spinal cord: pathway for neural fibers traveling to and from brain; controls simple reflexes

Cerebellum: coordinates voluntary movement and balance and supports memories of such

Amygdala: linked to emotion

Hippocampus: linked to memory

Right hemisphere

Left hemisphere

Cerebral cortex ▨ Limbic system ▨ Brainstem

Figure 4.2.

THE DIENCEPHALON: HYPOTHALAMUS AND THALAMUS

The diencephalon sits just above the midbrain and is made up of the *hypothalamus* and the *thalamus*. The hypothalamus is the brain's primary drive center. The three primary drives (eating, drinking and sex) are directed by the functioning of specialized nuclei (clusters of neurons) in the hypothalamus. These nuclei are clustered together and govern each drive. It is important to note that the sexual drive is located in the same region as the centers for eating and drinking. Thus the sexual/reproductive drive is experienced as a survival need similar to the drive for eating and drinking. However, while you can die from not eating or drinking, you can't really die from lack of sexual activity. The hypothalamus is connected with the pituitary gland and coordinates the release of the majority of the body's hormones such as cortisol stress hormones, growth hormone, reproductive hormones (testosterone, estrogen) and many others. Through this hormonal system, the brain coordinates the body's response to prepare it for action and monitor the body's internal state.

The second component of the diencephalon is the thalamus. The thalamus acts as the brain's sensory relay station. Vision, hearing, taste and touch signals from the eyes, ears, mouth and skin all stop off in the thalamus where they are then processed and sent along to the sensory cortex where we see, hear, taste and feel. Where the hypothalamus is primarily responsible for internal drives, the thalamus is responsible for coordinating the information coming in from the outside. The primary nucleus in the thalamus responsible for visual signals is the *lateral geniculate nucleus* (LGN). The LGN serves to sort out the visual signals coming in from the eye and prepares them for more complex processing. The LGN marks the first spot in the brain where visual sexual stimuli are processed. If the eyes are the gateway to the soul, the LGN is the eye's gateway to the brain. More flexible in adapting to challenges than the midbrain, the diencephalon is still better understood as a "hardwired" region showing limited plasticity.

TELENCEPHALON: LIMBIC SYSTEM,
BASAL GANGLIA AND CORTEX

Resting atop the thalamus is the second component of the forebrain, the *telencephalon*. The telencephalon is comprised of three major brain systems: the limbic system, the basal ganglia and the cortex. The *limbic system* is a network of regions that is connected with the diencephalon's hypothalamus. It has two major components, the *amygdala* and the *hippocampus*. The amygdala is the brain region that is involved in the expression of emotions and emotional learning. It sits nestled on both sides of the brain underneath the cortex (see Figure 4.2) and damage to it can result in emotional disruptions such as decreased emotionality, a lack of appropriate fear, and hypersexuality known as Klüver-Bucy syndrome. The amygdala is also known to be involved in many mood and anxiety disorders such as post-traumatic stress disorder (Shin, Rauch and Pitman, 2006, pp. 67-79). The drive tension generated by the hypothalamus sends signals to the amygdala where the tension is psychologically experienced.

Connected to the amygdala is the *hippocampus*. The hippocampus's primary role is to take sensory information and store this information as a memory, but it also is important for mapping out the world (i.e., spatial navigation). Death of cells or disruption of connections in the hippocampus can result in memory problems often seen in forms of dementia like Alzheimer's disease. The *basal ganglia* is situated adjacent to the amygdala and hippocampus, and is made up of two major regions, the *striatum* and the *globus pallidus*. Both are associated with a number of functions but are best known for their importance in motor control as the site of Parkinson's and Huntington's diseases.

Above the basal ganglia and limbic system is the thinking part of the brain, the *cortex*. The cortex is the wrinkled gray matter that sits on the outermost part of the brain. It is divided into four lobes (frontal, parietal, occipital and temporal), and each lobe is made up of several folded layers of cortex called *gyri*. Each lobe and gyrus performs specific tasks and functions. For example, the temporal lobe is involved in hearing and language, the occipital lobe in vision, the parietal lobe in touch and the frontal lobe in complex thought. Each part of the cortex is constantly adjusting its synapses, processing, planning and responding to our world. Much of our psychological experience emerges out of the cortex. The cortex is where our most complex thoughts arise and has inherently a greater level of flexibility enabling abstract thought, language, consciousness, virtue and vice.

Those are the basic components of the brain. Now let's examine what happens when pornography is consumed.

PROCESSING THE SEXUAL IMAGE

Visual perception can be understood neurologically as following a straightforward path. The eye picks up the visual signal and sends a neural signal to the LGN. This signal is then relayed to the visual cortex found in the occipital lobe at the back of the head. From here the basics of the stimulus are then processed (what is the stimulus and where is it in the environment). But here is where things get interesting, where pornographic images become "HD" signals.

Men viewing a nude woman spend more time looking at her body and less time at her face. The focus is on her bodily parts. She is an object to be viewed and consumed (Lykins, Meana and Kambe, 2006, pp. 569-75). But there does appear to be a difference when men look at just a naked woman versus a couple engaging in intercourse. Contrary to popular belief, men do not focus just on a woman's bodily parts when they view heterosexual intercourse (Rupp and Wallen, 2007, pp. 524-33). When viewing sexual intercourse, men still spend a significant amount of time looking at the woman's body, but they also spend time examining the woman's face, presumably looking for her response to the sexual act. Men are more preoccupied with a woman's sexual arousal than they are given credit for.

The visual cortex and its primary outputs are more active in men than in women when they view pornography (Bocher et al., 2001, pp. 105-17). There is an increase in hypothalamic and VTA activity, which is likely correlated to the release of dopamine fueling the salience of the sexual signals. A number of sites in the cortex are related to emotional drives and are affected by sexual arousal, activity and response. The *insular cortex* has many connections to limbic regions, has been identified as a center for bodily representation and provides the context for subjective emotional experiences. Increases in insular cortex activity are seen in men when they are exposed to pornographic material. It is where some of the craving and preoccupation with sexual arousal reside (likely fueled by dopamine release). The *orbitofrontal cortex* is another cortical region that is wired with limbic sites and it also increases its activity when viewing pornography. There is also a considerable increase in the ventral portion of the striatum (the site of much of the VTA's dopamine output) (Arnow et al., 2002, p. 1014).

When men view pornography, they experience increased anxiety and tension, resulting in an increase in amygdala activity. Men also show an increase in amygdala activity when shown statements suggesting sexual infidelity by their girlfriend. Sexual arousal and intimate sexual relationships appear to supercharge the male amygdala.

Several brain regions in men are affected by stimulation of the penis and orgasm. There is an increase in activity in the VTA and insular cortex, but there is a decrease in the activity of the amygdala. While the VTA and insula appear to be the sites responsible for the release of dopamine and the psychological experience of euphoria and transcendence. There is also a dramatic reduction in the activity of the amygdala. As sexual tension increases amygdala activity, the orgasm releases this tension and anxiety (Holstege et al., 2003, pp. 9185-93).

MIRROR NEURONS

Another significant finding in brain research is the presence of *mirror neurons*. Mirror neurons are a set of brain cells found in specific parts of the brain, notably the inferior frontal gyrus and the inferior parietal lobe (Mouras et al., 2008, pp. 1142-50). These neurons were thought to be only involved in the production of a behavior but are more than that. They're also involved in the *perception* of that same behavior. They are motor system cells that activate when you see a behavior. If you see someone grab a pen, neurons that would correspond to his or her grabbing a pen are activated in you as well. Originally called "monkey see, monkey do" neurons since they were first discovered in monkeys, these cells act as mirrors. When we see a behavior, we silently mirror it in our cortex. It's as if the cortex says "I can do that" and mirrors how it would actually do it.

Mirror neurons have been implicated in many other important fields like the study of observational learning and autism (Williams et al., 2001, p. 287; Malle and Hodges, 2005, p. 354). They are located in the same cortical regions that are involved in language development and detecting emotions in others. When you see the face of someone who is afraid, it elicits the same emotional state in you.

How are mirror neurons related to pornography? Consider what happens with mirror neurons when men watch a pornographic video. The brain reacts in such a way as if you were the person engaged in the sexual act. Viewing a pornographic movie creates a neurological experience whereby a person vicariously participates in what he is watching. As a man watches a pornographic movie he can neurologically identify with the performers in the video and place himself into the HD signal. No longer is he restricted to responding to just the nakedness of the woman. To deal with the arousal it creates, the brain mirrors and heightens the arousal, causing even more sexual tension. The sexual drive is fueled even further and screams for an outlet.

THE SEXUAL OUTLET OF CONVENIENCE
In another study of brain activation during human male ejaculation, researchers in the Netherlands discovered that when men are placed in a brain scanner and are stimulated by volunteer female partners, VTA activity increases as well. The VTA is known to have dopaminergic projections to a variety of forebrain structures. The structures, most notably in the nucleus accumbens and the cingulate cortex, have long been known to be involved in the neural circuitry of reward. This connection from the VTA to these limbic regions is the source of the rush from substances of abuse as well as sexual arousal. As researchers have suggested, "The present findings may represent an anatomi-

cal substrata for the strongly reinforcing nature of sexual activity in humans. Because ejaculation introduces sperm into the female reproductive tract, it would be critical for reproduction of the species to favor ejaculation as the most rewarding behavior" (Holstege et al., 2003, pp. 9185-93). This area also shows an increase in activation when cocaine and heroin are administered and is involved in rewarding behaviors such as eating and drinking.

A number of other regions are collectively referred to as the *mesodiencephalic transition zone*. This mesodiencephalic transition zone receives input from the spinal cord so that when the ejaculatory reflex occurs, it is accompanied by a signal sent to the brain that initiates the psychological experience of an orgasm. These connections go throughout the spinal cord, but particularly the region innervating the genitals in other species. Several regions of the cortex were found to be activated while other regions deactivated. The majority of the activation usually occurred on the right side of a brain, which is involved with memory-related inventory while the secondary visual cortex is involved in visual hallucinations. The researchers also noticed that there was an absence of activation in the medial preoptic area (MPOA) and amygdala of these males. The absence of MPOA activation (which in non-primates is incredibly important for arousal and ejaculation) seems to suggest that this region in humans is involved in creating the context for sexual behavior. The deactivation of the amygdala and entorhinal cortex is also seen in subjects who view pictures of loved ones as well as subjects who experience a cocaine rush.

These findings suggest that human ejaculation due to stimulation by a partner (or by oneself) correlates with the euphoric, orgasmic states that are seen in heroin and cocaine use. Because of this activity, many have referred to people being addicted to sex. The orbitofrontal cortex is our emotional modulatory system. This is our decision-making system. To be addicted to something is to release dopamine, which causes you to want it and to make the decision to pursue it. That's our addiction pathway.

What about watching pornography? Well, it comes in through the retina, goes through the thalamus, when projects up to the visual cortex, goes through the association cortex and the anterior cingulate, which then projects down to the insular cortex, the mirror neuron system, and the basal ganglia, thalamus and the hypothalamus. This is the sexual arousal center, that interstitial nucleus of the anterior hypothalamus that sends projections down to the ventral tegmental area, which then releases dopamine.

Watching sex increases sexual anxiety (myotonia). In an overactive and in a heightened state of emotional arousal, the myotonic state needs to be resolved. What is the easiest route to resolving the myotonia? Ejaculation. This network is why pornography is so insidious in males; it is not the same in females. Females are not aroused like males by visual images of pornography, but this doesn't mean the visual signal is unimportant, just *less* important than in males.

What happens in ejaculation? Usually there's some sort of stimulation coming from the spinal cord, which goes up to the hypothalamus. It also goes to the VTA, because when there's ejaculation, there's a release of dopamine. All this shuts down the amygdala. Why is that important? The amygdala is our emotional center and primarily our fear center in the brain. The amygdala shuts down at the moment of ejaculation. Thus an orgasm is associated with an absence of fear. Men experience a sort of emotional hovering, a transcendent freedom from all worry.

The caudate, the putamen and the pallidum (together the basal ganglia) are implicit learning centers. This is the site of unwritten rules. Consider these thought patterns: *If I scrub my hands, I'll make the anxiety about my dirtiness go away. If I scrub my hands, I'll feel clean. If I check the house, I'll know that the iron isn't on.* Some people know they've already checked the iron but can't get rid of the anxiety. The only way they can get it out of their head is to repeat the behavior involving the basal ganglia.

This leads us to a pathway that makes viewing pornography a seemingly pleasurable experience. Males like looking at pornography. Naked women are interesting and arousing. When sexual images come through the visual system they stimulate sexual arousal. When there is a male performer, they can (via the mirror neurons) vicariously participate in the sexual act. If they arouse themselves and masturbate to pornography, they now begin to set in place a neurological habit. The images, arousal, masturbatory act and ejaculation are all associated with one another.

This is how a pornography addiction and sexual compulsion is built from scratch. It involves the visual system (looking at porn), the motor system (masturbating), the sensory system (genital stimulation) and neurological effects of orgasm (sexual euphoria from opiates, addictive dopamine in the nucleus accumbens and reduced fear in the amygdale). They have now begun to store this pattern as a reinforced neurological habit.

THE CHEMICALS OF PASSION

Responses to pornography flow through the neurological viaducts through which feelings of love, longing, need and romance are experienced. These neurological circuits are the wires of the system, but there are other players as well. Hormones and neurotransmitters provide the "juice" within this wiring system. Understanding their roles in activating this system is critical. Let's consider some of the major hormonal and neurotransmitter substances that are major players in the brain and body's chemistry of love and sexual intimacy, with special attention to their role in men.

TESTOSTERONE

If any one hormone has the reputation as being the male hormone, it is testosterone. Often blamed for all that is considered bad masculine behavior, from aggression to dominance, it is also heralded as the magic elixir that promises to restore men to their virile, masculine selves. It plays a key role in sexual development, and in the adult it is important for sexual interest and motivation. The adult male produces about forty to sixty times more testosterone than a female, but testosterone levels can vary greatly between men. Testosterone affects the whole body, increases the size of many organs on average (such as lungs, liver and heart) and is involved in the masculinization of the brain during development (see chapter 6).

Testosterone is released into the bloodstream throughout the day, but is increased in response to sexual cues picked up by the brain. The brain detects these sexual cues and initiates an increased production of testosterone by the testes. This increase in testosterone feeds back to the brain, enhancing sexual anticipation and preparing the brain for further sexual stimuli. This increase in sexual cues can be produced from the outside (the presence of a potential partner or pornographic image) or from within (sexual fantasizing). While testosterone does not enhance sexual performance, it acts as the hormone driving sexual desire. This is why castration is used for the removal of the sexual drive (i.e., eunuchs and chemical castration for sex offenders).

The wave of testosterone, however, is slow to dissipate. It has an extended period of activation, unlike neurotransmitters, which have a much shorter duration time. Testosterone is the hormone that primes both the body and the brain in preparation for sexual intimacy. Pornography (and the mental fantasizing that it enables) crafts a brain that constantly generates testosterone and heightens sexual desire. With this ever-present sexual desire, the brain is ready to interpret any signal (external or internal) and ramp up the perceived need for sexual activity. Interestingly, men in committed relationships tend to have lower testosterone levels. This may be a reason why these men may be less likely to commit adultery (Burnham et al., 2003, pp. 119-22).

DOPAMINE

Dopamine is the neurotransmitter involved in the mesolimbic system that coordinates all natural reinforcing behaviors (eating, drinking, sex). It is also the primary neurotransmitter that most addictive drugs are known to release. Dopamine plays an important role in reinforcement and is part of the reason why craving occurs. Sometimes referred to as a pleasure chemical, dopamine focuses our attention on things that have significance to us. Eating a good meal when hungry, drinking a cool glass of water when thirsty or making love to your wife all have emotional salience. Dopamine helps us know where we should direct our energy. It is not surprising then that dopamine has been implicated in many other mental illnesses such as attention deficit disorder, obsessive-compulsive disorder and schizophrenia.

In the brain, dopamine is involved in movement (Parkinson's disease is an example of this; lack of dopamine results in an inability to move), but it is better known for its involvement in addiction. Dopamine is released into the specific brain regions (the limbic system's nucleus accumbens), but it is not where we experience "pleasure." The activation of dopamine receptors in this area involves how our arousal is directed and how the significance of our needs is determined. This stimulus we are attending to and experiencing is then stored in our memory (along with the consequences of the drug, image, lover, etc.) and prepares us for the next time the need wells up within us.

Sexual cues trigger the release of dopamine in the nucleus accumbens, which is also sensitive to testosterone. This synergy between dopamine and testosterone is such that the elevation of testosterone enhances dopamine's sex significance, and the elevation of dopamine activation propels testosterone levels. Convenient, isn't it? Dopamine focuses a man, initiates his movements, increases his sexual sensitivity and makes him long for his sexual partner.

NOREPINEPHRINE

Norepinephrine (sometimes known as noradrenaline) is a pharmacological switch-hitter. It can act as a hormone or as a neurotransmitter. It is also important in sexual arousal and sexual memory as a hormone and as a neurotransmitter. Norepinephrine is a chemical cousin of dopamine (together they are the *catecholamines*) and is also similar to epinephrine (or adrenaline). It is found throughout the brain and can act as a stress hormone involved in directing our responses to autonomic arousal (fight or flight, fear, anxiety, panic, excitement, sexual arousal). In autonomic arousal, norepinephrine and epinephrine (produced by the adrenal glands next to the kidneys) increase heart rate, trigger the release of sugar for energy and move the blood from our core to our muscles (for fight or flight). It is involved in alertness and waking you up from sleep (noradrenergic drugs can be stimulants to keep you awake). Epinephrine-based drugs have been used as appetite suppressants.

Important in the context of sexual arousal, norepinephrine and epinephrine are part of the autonomic arousal that occurs throughout the body in preparation for sexual activity. It is this autonomic arousal (specifically what is referred to as the sympathetic division of the autonomic nervous system) that gives some the feeling of being ramped up or energized. However, this autonomic activation is not directed.

A person can be energized in many ways. He can be energized at the prospect of a meal when hungry, for a drink when thirsty or for a sexual encounter. He can also be energized to run away from a fight, avoid a predator, engage in a fight, prepare for an athletic event or cheer on his favorite team. Sometimes our world forces us into arousal (when we are attacked or when we see pornography). Other times we work ourselves into an aroused state (we dwell on an injustice or we fantasize). Regardless of how a man gets aroused, his brain is involved in making sense of the arousal and determining how to respond to it.

When I took my son to an art museum, he saw some paintings of nudes. The images created an autonomic arousal that he had no context to interpret, so he giggled. But in an older man who has been informed about the place of sexuality and nakedness and has a sexual history, the arousal is interpreted as sexual. The neurological process that he has learned is initiated. If he has a history of acting out in an unhealthy manner, he will most likely do so again and reinforce the process. If he has a history of directing his arousal in a healthy fashion, he will most likely do so again and continue the process of sanctification. Norepinephrine is the hormone that initiates the arousal in our body and creates the sense of energy, however we interpret it.

In the brain norepinephrine is also involved in storing emotional stimuli. It has been implicated in the formation of flashbulb memories and post-traumatic stress disorder. Norepinephrine burns the object that initiated the arousal into our memories because of its physiological and emotional significance. Is it any wonder why so many men can pull up clear memories of uninvited pornographic images that they were exposed to when they were young? Is it any wonder why they have been scarred in a PTSD-like fashion, unable to erase these images? And is it any wonder why men who act out in response to pornography often have these images return (both uninvited and invited) with such ease? We were designed to store significant experiences of sexual intimacy with norepinephrine's help.

SEROTONIN

The use of the antidepressant Prozac and the illegal drug ecstasy have popularized the neurotransmitter serotonin as the brain chemical involved in mood and emotional euphoria. It is true that increased levels of serotonin help people who are depressed, but one of their most notorious side effects is sexual dysfunction. By increasing serotonin levels to elevate mood, there is a decrease in the sexual response of men. Low levels of serotonin in women may make them more likely to become depressed, but in men low serotonin is more likely to make them impulsive and aggressive. This may seem a bit odd; increasing a mood elevator should enhance sexual mood, shouldn't it? But as seen in the use of the street drug ecstasy, why have sex when the high you get off of the drug is better? (Ecstasy works with other neurotransmitter systems to produce this euphoria.) By increasing serotonin levels, interest in sex is diminished. Combined with the fact that dopamine tends to suppress serotonin, reduced levels of serotonin seem to be important for sexual arousal.

ENDOGENOUS OPIATES

The rush that a man gets from seeing an attractive woman is different from the rush he gets from an orgasm. The chemical difference between these two is that sexual arousal is the result of testosterone, dopamine and norepinephrine surges, whereas the transcendence and euphoria experienced during orgasm is related to the release of endogenous opiates. The body produces natural or endogenous opiates involved in pain relief and reinforcement. Artificial drugs like heroine cause euphoria and reduce pain distress. This may be why many men describe the psychological and emotional aspects of orgasm as a "release." The ejaculatory release of semen occurs in concert with opiate activation (Holstege et al., 2003, pp. 9185-93; Moulier et al., 2006, pp. 689-99; Holstege, 2005, pp. 109-14).

The resulting opiate release and orgasm also is connected with two other systems: dopamine release in the nucleus accumbens and decreased amygdala activity. Because of the nature of the wiring, spinal signals arriving from the body that are connected with ejaculation release opiates onto the site which is the primary source of dopamine to the nucleus accumbens—VTA. The amygdala and cingulate cortex interpret the autonomic arousal as fear or anxiety, sometimes referred to in a sexual context as sexual tension.

The movement toward orgasm in men is usually accompanied by an increased state of anxiety. One man once described it to me as a "pre-orgasmic panic." But this elevation in amygdala activity is shut off as a result of the opiate being released with ejaculation. The opiates' activation resulting from ejaculation increases the amount of dopamine released in the VTA and shuts down the fear-based amygdala. This adds significance and pleasure to the euphoria and the removal of all fear.

But the male mind is not made to achieve this orgasmic high on demand. Considerable neurological work goes into preparing a brain for an endogenous release of opiates. It is designed to be preceded by the priming of dopamine, norepinephrine and testosterone. However, repeated activation of opiate receptors (such as with heroin addiction or repeated orgasm) results in tolerance. With repeated acting out (as well as drug use), the absence of opiate activation results in craving (the drug or sexual release) and diminished euphoria. This is why coupling pornography with masturbation is so significant in the development of pornography problems and ultimately steals the joy from sexual relations.

OXYTOCIN AND VASOPRESSIN

If testosterone gets desire started, oxytocin and vasopressin are what bind men to the object of their affection. Oxytocin and vasopressin are released slowly during sexual activity, but are released in large quantities in response to orgasm. Oxytocin is released in the brain and is detected in several parts of the brain that are implicated in the qualitative experience of sexual satisfaction, such as amygdala, ventromedial hypothalamus and septum (Murphy et al., 1987). Comparative studies of the effects of oxytocin on males indicate that it is involved in erection and that vasopressin released in the brain of males after sexual intercourse increases their social attachment to their partner. In nonsexual experiments, men who are administered oxytocin display a higher level of trust and a reduction of fear in risky situations when compared to non-oxytocin controls. When a man plays a game against a computer opponent, the presence of oxytocin did nothing to create trust or reduce his aversion to risk, indicating that it is about attachment and trust in a person and not the situation (Kosfeld et al., 2005).

Vasopressin is released in the brain during sexual behavior and is particularly important in binding the male to his mate. There is also some indication that vasopressin may be involved in protecting the mate and becoming aggressive toward other males. One study has gone so far as to argue that a gene which codes for vasopressin receptors has been correlated with marital status, marital bonding, and the spouse's perception of marital quality. Unfortunately, with repeated sexual acting out in the absence of a partner, a man will be bound and attached to the image and not a person.

While a man may have many reasons for viewing pornography, the act of viewing activates the mirror system and increases the need for orgasm/ejaculation (usually via masturbation or sexually acting out). When this occurs, this maladaptive pattern is neurologically and neurochemically reinforced.

FROM PORNOGRAPHIC TROUGH TO SANCTIFIED WIRING

When I was young I visited a farm that had an old-fashioned water pump. It was situated in the center of a cement slab and would drip ferociously, long after you stopped pumping. Over the years the left-over dripping water had cut a trough from under the spigot to the edge of the slab. The trough was nearly two inches deep, and any standing water on the slab would be channeled to it, cutting it deeper.

So it is with pornography in a man's brain. Because of the way that the male brain is wired, it is prone to pick up on sexually relevant cues. These cues trigger arousal and a series of neurological, hormonal and neurochemical events are set into motion. Memories about how to respond to these cues are set off and the psychological, emotional and behavioral response begins. As the pattern of arousal and response continues, it deepens the neurological pathway, making a trough.

This neural system trough, along with neurotransmitters and hormones, are the underlying physical realities of a man's sexual experience. Each time that an unhealthy sexual pattern is repeated, a neurological, emotional and spiritual erosion carves out a channel that will eventually develop into a canyon from which there is no escape.

But if this corrupted pathway can be avoided, a new pathway can be formed. We can establish a healthy sexual pattern where the flow is redirected toward holiness rather than corrupted intimacy. By intentionally redirecting the neurochemical flow, the path toward right thinking becomes the preferred path and is established as the mental habit. The path to recovery relies on the very rules that govern how the wounds were initially created. By deepening the "holiness" pathways, we are freed from deciding to do what is right and good as they become part of our embodied nature. That is part of the process of sanctification.

REFERENCES

Andersen, S. L., and M. H. Teicher. 2000. Sex differences in dopamine receptors and their relevance to ADHD. *Neuroscience and Biobehavioral Reviews* 24, no. 1: 137-41.

Ariely, D., and G. Loewenstein. 2006. The heat of the moment: the effect of sexual arousal on sexual decision making. *Journal of Behavioral Decision Making* 19, no. 2: 87.

Arnold, A. P. 2004. Sex chromosomes and brain gender. *Nature reviews. Neuroscience* 5, no. 9 (Sep): 701-8.

Arnow, B. A., J. E. Desmond, L. L. Banner, G. H. Glover, A. Solomon, M. L. Polan, T. F. Lue, and S. W. Atlas. 2002. Brain activation and sexual arousal in healthy, heterosexual males. *Brain* 125, no. 5: 1014.

Baron-Cohen, S., S. Lutchmaya and R. Knickmeyer. 2004. *Prenatal testosterone in mind: Amniotic fluid studies.* Cambridge, MA: The MIT Press.

Berridge, K. C. 2007. The debate over dopamine's role in reward: the case for incentive salience. *Psychopharmacology* 191, no. 3: 391-431.

Berridge, K. C., and P. Winkielman. 2003. What is an unconscious emotion? (The case for unconscious 'liking'.). *Cognition and Emotion* 17, no. 2: 181-211.

Biderman, Irving, and Edward A. Vessel. 2006. Perceptual pleasure and the brain. *American Scientist* 94 (3): 247-53.

Biederman, Joseph, and Stephen V. Faraone. 2006. Attention-deficit hyperactivity disorder. *The Lancet* 366, no. 9481: 237-48.

Bitran, D., and E. M. Hull. 1987. Pharmacological analysis of male rat sexual behavior. *Neuroscience and biobehavioral reviews* 11, no. 4: 365-89.

Bocher, M., R. Chisin, Y. Parag, N. Freedman, Y. Meir Weil, H. Lester,

E. Mishani and O. Bonne. 2001. Cerebral activation associated with sexual arousal in response to a pornographic clip: A 15O–H2O PET study in heterosexual men. *NeuroImage* 14, no. 1: 105-17.

Bowling, Shana L., James K. Rowlett and Michael T. Bardo. 1993. The effect of environmental enrichment on amphetamine-stimulated locomotor activity, dopamine synthesis and dopamine release. *Neuropharmacology* 32, no. 9: 885-93.

Brizendine, L. 2006. *The female brain*. New York: Random House.

Burnham, T. C., J. F. Chapman, P. B. Gray, M. H. McIntyre, S. F. Lipson and P. T. Ellison. 2003. Men in committed, romantic relationships have lower testosterone. *Hormones and Behavior* 44, no. 2 (8): 119-22.

Cahill, L. 2006. *Why sex matters for neuroscience*. England Nature Pub. Group.

Castellanos, F. X., Paul E. A. Glaser and Greg A. Gerhardt. 2006. Towards a neuroscience of attention-deficit/hyperactivity disorder: Fractionating the phenotype. *Journal of Neuroscience Methods* 151, no. 1 (2/15): 1-4.

Dalley, Jeffrey W., Adam C. Mar, Daina Economidou and Trevor W. Robbins. 2008. Neurobehavioral mechanisms of impulsivity: Fronto-striatal systems and functional neurochemistry. *Pharmacology Biochemistry and Behavior*.

Hakyemez, Hélène S., Alain Dagher, Stephen D. Smith and David H. Zald. 2008. Striatal dopamine transmission in healthy humans during a passive monetary reward task. *NeuroImage* 39, no. 4 (2/15) : 2058-65.

Holstege, G. 2005. Central nervous system control of ejaculation. *World Journal of Urology* 23, no. 2 (Jun): 109-14.

Holstege, G., J. R. Georgiadis, A. M. Paans, L. C. Meiners, F. H. van der Graaf and A. A. Reinders. 2003. Brain activation during human male ejaculation. *Journal of Neuroscience* 23, no. 27 (Oct 8): 9185-93.

Janssen, E., D. Carpenter and C. A. Graham. 2003. Selecting Films for Sex Research: Gender Differences in Erotic Film Preference. *Ar-

chives of Sexual Behavior 32, no. 3: 243-51.

Kakade, Sham, and Peter Dayan. 2002. Dopamine: generalization and bonuses. *Neural Networks* 15, no. 4-6: 549-59.

Karama, S., A. R. Lecours, J. M. Leroux, P. Bourgouin, G. Beaudoin, S. Joubert and M. Beauregard. 2002. Areas of brain activation in males and females during viewing of erotic film excerpts. *Human Brain Mapping* 16, no. 1, pp. 1-13 (1 p.1/2).

Kosfeld, Michael, Markus Heinrichs, Paul J. Zak, Urs Fischbacher and Ernst Fehr. 2005. Oxytocin increases trust in humans. *Nature* 435: 673-76.

Koukounas, Eric, and Marita McCabe. 1997. Sexual and emotional variables influencing sexual response to erotica. *Behaviour Research and Therapy* 35, no. 3 (3): 221-30.

Krain, Amy L., and F. X. Castellanos. 2006. Brain development and ADHD. *Clinical Psychology Review,* 26, no. 4 (8): 433-444.

Krause, Klaus-Henning, Stefan H. Dresel, Johanna Krause, Christian la Fougere, and Manfred Ackenheil. 2003. The dopamine transporter and neuroimaging in attention deficit hyperactivity disorder. *Neuroscience & Biobehavioral Reviews,* 27, no. 7 (11): 605-13.

Lykins, A. D., M. Meana and G. Kambe. 2006. Detection of differential viewing patterns to erotic and non-erotic stimuli using eye-tracking methodology. *Archives of Sexual Behavior* 35, no. 5 (Oct): 569-75.

Malle, Bertram F., and Sara D. Hodges. 2005. *Other minds: How humans bridge the divide between self and others.* New York: Guilford Press.

McCabe, D. P., and A. D. Castel. 2008. Seeing is believing: The effect of brain images on judgments of scientific reasoning. *Cognition* 107, no. 1: 343-352.

Melis, M. R., and A. Argiolas. 1995. Dopamine and sexual behavior. *Neuroscience and biobehavioral reviews* 19, no. 1: 19-38.

Moulier, V., H. Mouras, M. Pélégrini-Issac, D. Glutron, R. Rouxel, B. Grandjean, J. Bittoun and S. Stoléru. 2006. Neuroanatomical correlates of penile erection evoked by photographic stimuli in human males. *NeuroImage* 33, no. 2 (Nov 1): 689-99.

Mouras, H., S. Stoléru, V. Moulier, M. Pélégrini-Issac, R. Rouxel, B. Grandjean, D. Glutron and J. Bittoun. 2008. Activation of mirror-neuron system by erotic video clips predicts degree of induced erection: an MRI study. *NeuroImage* 42, no. 3: 1142-50.

Murphy M. E., J. R. Seckl, S. Burton, S. A. Checkley and S. L. Lightman. 1987. "Changes in oxytocin and vasopressin secretion during sexual activity in men" *Journal of Clinical Endocrinology and Metabolism* 65: 738-41.

Rupp, H. A., and K. Wallen. 2007. Sex differences in viewing sexual stimuli: An eye-tracking study in men and women. *Hormones and behavior* 51, no. 4: 524-33.

Russell, Vivienne A. 2007. Neurobiology of animal models of attention-deficit hyperactivity disorder. *Journal of Neuroscience Methods* 161, no. 2 (4/15): 185-98.

Shin, L. M., S. L. Rauch, and R. K. Pitman. 2006. Amygdala, medial prefrontal cortex, and hippocampal function in PTSD. *Annals of the New York Academy of Sciences* 1071, no. 1. Psychobiology of Posttraumatic Stress Disorder: A Decade of Progress: 67-79.

Sikström, Sverker, Göran Söderlund. 2007. Stimulus-Dependent Dopamine Release in Attention-Deficit/Hyperactivity Disorder. *Psychological Review* 114, no. 4 (10): 1047-75.

Ströhle, Andreas, Meline Stoy, Jana Wrase, Steffi Schwarzer, Florian Schlagenhauf, Michael Huss, Jakob Hein, Anke Nedderhut, Britta Neumann, Andreas Gregor, Georg Juckel, Brian Knutson, Ulrike Lehmkuhl, Michael Bauer and Andreas Heinz. 2008. Reward anticipation and outcomes in adult males with attention-deficit/hyperactivity disorder. *NeuroImage* 39, no. 3 (2/1): 966-72.

Utter, Amy A., and Michele A. Basso. 2008. The basal ganglia: An overview of circuits and function. *Neuroscience & Biobehavioral Reviews* 32, no. 3: 333-32.

van Furth, W. R., G. Wolterink and J. M. van Ree. 1995. Regulation of masculine sexual behavior: involvement of brain opiods and dopamine. *Brain Research Reviews* 21: 162-84.

Volkow, N. D., G. J. Wang, L. Maynard, M. Jayne, J. S. Fowler, W. Zhu, J. Logan, S. J. Gatley, Y. S. Ding and C. Wong. 2003. Brain dopamine is associated with eating behaviors in humans. *International Journal of Eating Disorders* 33, no. 2.

Williams, J. H. G., A. Whiten, T. Suddendorf and D. I. Perrett. 2001. *Imitation, mirror neurons and autism.* New York: Pergamon.

Part Two. **Healthy Masculinity & Sexuality**

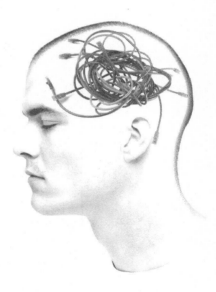

5

Made Male in God's Image

WHAT WE THINK ABOUT HOW WE ARE MADE affects every aspect of our life: what we can become, what we are capable of, what we are meant for, who we can love and what our limitations are. One underlying problem for many men is not pornography, but a wrong understanding of how they are made. They think of themselves as a soul trapped inside a body, enslaved to it. The soul is who they really are, not their body. Many think of the body as a shell that temporarily contains the soul and subjects it to base desires, wants and needs. The soul and the body are at war with each other, the soul longing for the good and the body craving the bad.

Many men believe that this soul is immortal and that if they want to live a good and holy life they must constantly battle against the evil cravings of the body. But is this a naïve view of our nature? Is it scripturally accurate? And does it fit with the findings of contemporary brain science? In order to understand our sexuality, we first have to address our humanity.

THEOLOGY: THREE VIEWS

What does it mean to be created in the image of God? In the Judeo Christian traditions, the *imago Dei* is found in three places in the book of Genesis. It appears first in the account of God creating man in Genesis 1:26-27:

> Then God said, "Let us make man in our image, after our likeness. And let them have dominion over the fish of the sea and

over the birds of the heavens and over the livestock and over all the earth and over every creeping thing that creeps on the earth."

So God created man in his own image,
in the image of God he created him;
male and female he created them.

The Hebrew *tselem* is translated into *imago* in Latin and into English as "image." The Hebrew *demuth* is translated into the Latin as *similtudo* and into English as "likeness." These terms image and likeness appear a few chapters later, where they are switched in order and refer to Adam's fathering of Seth: "he fathered a son in his own likeness, after his image" (Gen 5:3). Later in Genesis 9 the "image" returns, but this time it bears a warning that communicates humanity's privileged and sacred position. "Whoever sheds the blood of man, by man shall his blood be shed, for God made man in his own image" (Gen 9:6). Because we bear the image of God, human life has an inviolable, sacred property. Humankind is to be treated in a manner that is different from the rest of creation. Systematically teasing out what *imago Dei* means has been a daunting task for many theologians. Theologians have understood *imago Dei* in several different ways (Hoekema, 1986).

THE IMAGE OF GOD AS SOUL

The first category of understanding the image of God is as *soul*. Perhaps the best example of this view of the image of God is seen in the substance dualism of the 17th century French philosopher Rene Descartes. Descartes argued that there are two fundamental kinds of substance: mental and material. According to this view, mental substances (like the soul) do not exist in time and space but are capable of thinking. The other substance, physical matter (the body), exists in time and space, and material cannot think. This type of substance dualism is compatible with a substance view of *imago Dei*—human beings are mental and material, body and soul. Descartes' philosophy was embraced by many in Western Christianity and has provided the foundation of philosophical thinking about humanity in Western thought for over 200 years. The soul leaves the body when we die.

This view, however, can also lead to some unintended negative consequences. We believe that each person is essentially comprised of an inner, nonmaterial part that defines who we truly are. For many Christians the state of our inner, nonmaterial soul is of the utmost importance. The soul is what lives on after the death of the body and is either rewarded with heaven or punished with damnation. For those who do not have a religious framework, the soul can be replaced by a mind, a self, or the "real me." New Age thought and contemporary mysticism have inherited this notion, but it can be found in many religious systems other than Christianity.

Substance dualism is not the only way that philosophers have conceptualized human nature, but it is the predominant one in our culture. There are many other philosophical systems that differ from substance dualism (Hoekema, 1986), but substance dualism forms the foundation for the way that many men think about how they are made: a Gnostic view of the body as bad. Their sexuality is closely associated with the body, and our souls need to be saved from our bodies.

THE IMAGE OF GOD AS FUNCTIONAL

The *functional view* holds that the image of God is manifest in human beings as they act as his representatives in this world. We act as God's agents in this world and that is our function. We image God as we perform our functions: being fruitful and multiplying, filling the earth, subduing and having dominion over the fish of the sea and birds of the air on God's behalf (Gen 1:28). The functional image is also known as the "political" image or cultural mandate, which emphasizes the governing or regency role that we have to explore and subdue creation. It points to our role as stewards, discoverers and cocreators within God's creation. We are the created vessels through which God is present in creation.

Many psychologists have grasped the notion of human uniqueness and have sought to understand how our minds work. In light of
this, psychologists tend to put human beings at the top of the heap
(as do theologians). By focusing on our powers of thought or emotion, morality or culture, psychologists have set up capacities as our
defining feature. We are rational, use language, play, worship, make
moral decisions, have complex social networks, are conscious and
intelligent. Unfortunately, whenever a cognitive or behavioral goal-
post is used to define our humanity, our non-human animal friends
find a way of qualifying. Monkeys can be rational, wolves show an
understanding of good and bad behavior, dolphins have complex
language skills, otters play. The result is that the psychologist feels
the need to move the goalposts back another 10 yards to soothe our
wounded species' ego.

The most recent addition to the game is the standard of culture.
This set of information, or memes, is passed from generation to generation, from societal member to societal member, providing a sort of
information-processing survival of the fittest. The pieces of information, these memes, procreate by being communicated via language
and birthed in the "mind" of the recipient. The capacity for abstract
thought, highly complex language, and coherent internal representation of the external world is created. From here we construct meaning
and purpose.

THE IMAGE OF GOD AS RELATIONAL

Some contemporary theologians such as Karl Barth have argued that
the image of God is better understood as *relational* in nature (Barth,
1977). This is seen in the Genesis 1:26 passage, "let us make man in
our image." The emphasis on "us" and "our" is a sign of joint activity
and relationality. This passage is early scriptural evidence of God's
triune nature, and this relational character has been transmitted from
God to humanity. This view sees the image of God's relational nature
in that human beings are in relationship with God, each other and
nature. The image may be best understood as humanity's special rela-

tionship with God, but is also present in our relationship with other people. Because of our finitude, consciousness, agency and embodiment, an "I-Thou" relationship will always exist with God and others. The image is seen in our relationships, especially with God. The relational view argues that bearing the image of God requires one to be in relationship with him. This relational capacity is best seen in our sexuality, the interaction of male and female, which together constitute the image of God.

Regardless of which perspective is taken, the original image of God was corrupted by the Fall and perverted. It is the state that we are born into. But it is through the sacrifice of Christ on the cross that humanity can be redeemed and renewed. Those who accept the gospel are then freed to be sanctified and perfected. It is important to not lose sight of this. Every man and every woman, all of humanity, can be seen in light of redemption and sanctification. The image of God can be seen in each person, but it also can be seen corporately in all of humanity.

Scripture does not speak about humanity in scientific terms. There are several ways of understanding what it means to be human, from theological doctrines of *imago Dei* and philosophical dualism to psychological theories of personhood, theory of mind and the self. In contrast with these approaches, a biological approach can range from genetic (having the right combinations of genes to make a human body) to neurological explanations (having the right kind of functioning brain). This emphasis on genetics, body and neurology is the hallmark of the biological understanding of humanity. I believe that moving away from the soul-based model of human uniqueness toward an *imago Dei*-based model rooted in relationality has more strength from philosophical, theological, biblical and scientific standpoints.

EMBODIMENT

The neurobiologist emphasizes the concept of embodiment. Embodiment means that we exist in a certain place and time and that we have a physical body that is necessary for our existence. Neurobiologists draw attention to studies that show that all of the theological, philosophical and psychological perspectives about human nature and uniqueness can be explained as a function of our brain activity (Brown, Murphy and Malony, 1998; Jeeves, 2004). The complex interplay in our neurological systems means that not only do neurons affect what is known, what is known affects the neurons. Christian theology makes clear that humankind is set apart from the rest of creation, and the question is whether or not it is a matter of degree or a matter of kind. Are we just a bit farther along with respect to a cognitive capacity? Are we just a little ahead of the curve, so to speak, when compared to the rest of creation? Or are we something that is just fundamentally different down to our core—not just quantitatively different, but qualitatively different?

A fear in many Christian circles is that if we lose the notion of the soul and reduce ourselves to physical substance and a mechanistic view of human nature, we lose what makes us unique. If there is no distinct substance that exists after death, then the only thing that matters is "matter." Similarly, if we are reduced to a thing (even a very complex and highly evolved thing), we lose any special place within creation. We have no greater value because we are made up of and are subject to the same laws as the rest of the physical universe.

The notion of emergence provides a way for neurons to come together in extraordinarily complex ways and produce our psychological experience (i.e., thoughts). These thoughts can then work backward (or downward) in the system and change structure and synapses of the brain. These structural changes then have functional significance as the brain feeds back, evaluates intentions, modifies actions, and reorganizes itself. With emergence a nesting of neural circuits within the brain provides a way for the neural brain to have hypercomplex feedback circuits and emerge as psychological experience.

Understanding a person as embodied with the emergence of psychological states is significant when we consider *imago Dei*. The principles of embodiment and emergence acknowledge our sexual nature and allow for it to extend beyond the function of reproduction. Our sexual longings can be about more than procreation; they can drive us toward intimacy with another human being and offer a taste of the transcendence found when we are in communion with God. Just as our needs for food, water, clothing and shelter point us toward the deeper needs whereby God sustains, covers and protects us, our sexuality also points us toward God as the one who meets our needs for intimacy and transcendence.

Just as the need for sustenance may be satisfied after a meal or drink, so the needs for intimacy and transcendence may be met when a husband and wife come together sexually. But eating, drinking and making love will only meet our needs for the moment; they will return. Only God is unchanging. We will be forever in a state of cyclical need as we eat, digest and then become hungry again. So because of our embodied nature, our need for intimacy and transcendence builds, is satisfied and then begins to slowly build again as we are separated from our beloved.

HUMAN BECOMINGS

The critical issue is not that we are just human beings, but what we are becoming—what is our purpose. While we are unified individual humans, we are also simultaneously being transformed, sometimes passively, sometimes actively, into something different. Human life is not static. We do not establish a homeostatic state and then maintain it indefinitely. Human life is an ongoing dynamic process where we begin as a fertilized egg, are implanted, develop *in utero*, are delivered, are nourished, cared for and challenged. We develop linguistic abilities and abstract symbolic systems. We adopt cognitive sets and meet environmental challenges through social embeddedness in our culture. We ask similar yet unique questions necessary for survival, making sense of the world as we are constantly changing and adapting, becoming something that we have not been.

This process of becoming is unique for each person but should be directed toward sanctification as we each uniquely are conformed to the image of Christ. Philip Hefner writes,

> For Christians the image of God is instantiated normatively in
> Jesus. Although this assertion has had a long and rich tradition
> of interpretation, there is no consensus on exactly what it means;
> there is no single official or even standard interpretation of the
> concept of the image of God. (Gregersen, Drees and Görman,
> 2000, p. 88)

The image of God is not a soulish substance, cognitive property,
behavioral function or capacity. To treat it as something to be identified, found or located is to miss the point. The Image of God is a
person: Jesus Christ. Colossians 1:15 states, "He [Jesus] is the image
of the invisible God, the firstborn of all creation." And 2 Corinthians
4:4 says, "In their case the god of this world has blinded the minds of
the unbelievers, to keep them from seeing the light of the gospel of the
glory of Christ, who is the image of God."

How are we made? To be made in the image of God is to be embodied and embedded in the story of creation. What is our purpose? Romans 8:29: "For those whom he foreknew he also predestined to be
conformed to the image of his Son, in order that he might be the firstborn among many brothers." Our purpose is to be conformed to the
image of Christ in how we live, breathe, think, act, worship and glo-
rify God. This involves our bodies.

Being made in the image of God is one of the foundational theological starting points that those in the Christian faith begin with
when examining humanity's place in the universe. It is because of our
"image-of-God-ness" that we believe that each human life is sacred.
We act as his agents and representatives in this world. Because of this
image we are interconnected to each other, relating with each other
and the Creator.

We live in a world that values others based on what they have accomplished in life, how intelligent they are or what their social status
is. But for the Christian, this is not where a person receives their value.
The value and dignity of each human life, male and female, is based

on the biblical doctrine that each person is made in the image of God. Our value is not in our intellectual abilities, social status, the number of children we produce, the number of degrees we obtain or the size of our bank account. Our value is found first in Christ Jesus, whose image we bear. It is not a matter of degree; it is categorical.

But life is not just about *being*; it is also about *becoming*. God's plan for us is that we become conformed to the image of Christ. This is the process of sanctification; it is what we are meant for. And human beings are not androgynous, sexless souls trapped in sexed bodies. Human beings are souls that are sexed as part of their embodied nature. Consider the famous quote by C. S. Lewis,

> It is a serious thing . . . to remember that the dullest and most uninteresting person you talk to may one day be a creature which, if you saw it now, you would be strongly tempted to worship, or else a horror and a corruption such as you now meet, if at all, only in a nightmare. All day long we are, in some degree, helping each other to one or the other of these destinations. It is in light of these overwhelming possibilities, it is with the awe and the circumspection proper to them, that we should conduct all our dealings with one another. . . . It is immortals whom we joke with, work with, marry, snub, and exploit—immortal horrors or everlasting splendors. (Lewis, 1977, pp. 14-15)

MADE MALE

Part of our embodiment is that we have reproductive anatomy. What is it that makes us male? What is it that makes a man? Is an adult male a man? Or is being a man more than just about being able to make babies? The distinction between male (which is a term used to address reproductive organs) and man (a term used more broadly usually to refer to an adult male who is spiritually, emotionally and psychologically mature) is critical. I know many adult males who have not yet matured to the point where they can leave home and hold down a job, pay their rent, wash their clothes or have a conversation with a woman without mentally undressing her. Many of us frown and talk about such males as not having "grown up" or being "not quite a man yet."

For most academics, sex refers to our reproductive categorization; it is a biological term. Gender refers to something beyond our reproductive organs; it refers to our psychological status. Because of this I think it is important that we make a distinction between the concept of maleness and manhood, between function and purpose. Maleness is a biological state dictated by the development of reproductive organs. Manhood is a sociological, psychological and spiritual state which is entered into. We often use the terms interchangeably, but the difference is important. We are often unaware of how the transition from our genetics to our psychological experience plays out, but when we look at it more closely we can see where changes in trajectory start to appear (Berenbaum, Korman and Leveroni, 1995, pp. 303-21; Chivers and Bailey, 2005, pp. 115-20; Mealey, 2000; Rahman, 2005, p. 1057).

REPRODUCTION

Reproductive ability, which is part of all life, is far-reaching and more complex than most of us give it credit for being. Sexual reproduction is not just for human beings; it is not what sets us apart from the rest of God's creation. The way we develop as sexual beings is however critically important. Being male or female impacts the way in which we think of ourselves, the social roles we play and the strengths and weaknesses that our bodies have even in the non-reproductive aspects of life (of which there are many).

Perhaps the most obvious thing that makes males and females distinct sexes is seen in their bodies. These distinct bodies (sometimes referred to as dimorphisms) can be easy to recognize. Whenever there is a dimorphism, there is (by definition) an inherent difference. The level of dimorphism in humans is not near as much as seen in other species (such as the colorful male peacock's plumage), but there are some obvious differences in humans (such as the genitalia, breasts in women, and on average men being larger) that are not difficult to spot.

In addition to these obvious differences between males and females are other differences that are less clear. These differences may be less in how organs may look and more in how they function. One organ where the majority of our cognitive and behavioral differences are rooted is that which yields our psychological experience: the brain. The interconnections in the brain are what underlie how we experience, feel and act in the world. It allows us to be conscious, to remember and to do most everything. It is fully integrated with the rest of the organs of the body and is in a constant neurological and hormonal dialogue with them.

THE MALE BRAIN

Research in the area of differences between male and female brains has been around for quite some time. For nearly fifty years the scientific community has been examining differences between not only the morphology or size of different brain regions but also the different ways in which these brains function. Research extends back to the 1950s on both humans and animals, looking at everything from learning to sexual behavior. Most of this research was done in adult animals, as there was an emphasis on finding out how the brains of males and females (which look similar, although the male brain is slightly larger) differ (Einstein, 2007).

So it's not a big surprise that men and women are different. But even today it is important to reaffirm that *different doesn't always mean superior or inferior.* Yes, men and women are different, but differences on any test or measure should never be used to infer greater or lesser value on the life of another human being. Remember, the image of God in each human being, male or female, gives them inherent worth and makes their life sacred. Women are not more valuable because they can have babies. Men are not more valuable because they have more muscle mass. Women are not more valuable because they may have greater verbal skills or larger vocabularies than men. Men are not more valuable because they can mentally rotate objects better than women. There may be times when such differences may be advantageous, but these differences are a matter of degree. Vocabulary, mental rotation, emotional sensitivity and intelligence are on a continuum, not all-or-nothing categories.

Just because a research study has found that there are statistical differences between males and females does not mean that these differences should be translated to all people in all circumstances. While it may be true that the average score of males may be higher than females on some tasks, it does not mean that every male is better than every female on that task. Just because I am a male does not mean that I'm better than every woman on the face of the planet when it comes to the mental rotation of three-dimensional objects. The truth be told, I'm actually not very good at those tasks. In the same way, some females are not nearly as verbal or have as large a vocabulary as some of my male colleagues. While females may score better on average on a language task, it does not mean that every female is better than every male on language tasks. So whenever considering the differences between males and females, it is important to remember that we're talking about averages. That being said, sometimes these differences play out in significant ways in real life.

TRAJECTORY

So what happens when males and females perform differently on a particular task? Sometimes it may be important, and sometimes it may not be. When I was growing up, my father and I were trying to fine-tune a scope on a rifle. My dad had attached the scope on the rifle and set up a can on a log approximately thirty yards away. When I took my first shot, I aimed for the center of the can and I succeeded in knocking it off the log. My dad looked at the can and then moved it another twenty yards away, setting it on a stump. When I aimed at the center of the can the second time and fired, nothing happened. The can remain on the stump. I had missed it. My dad adjusted the scope and then asked me to try again. When I fired the third time at the center of the can, I missed again. After another adjustment, my next round struck the can and knocked it off of the log.

The further away I moved from the target, the more important those few degrees of difference became. The difference between where the rifle's barrel was pointed and where the scope was focused was negligible when the target was close. But when the target was more distant, that small degree of difference between the scope and the barrel proved to be significant.

Sometimes these small degrees of difference dictate whether you hit or miss the target. When the can is close, the small difference may not impact the target being hit. There may be some slight differences in preferred styles of accomplishing those tasks but they are negligible. But there are times when these differences are important and the end result may be a missed target.

As our brains are knit together, men are predisposed to some behaviors and thought patterns, and females to others. How does this occur? One's sex affects their thoughts, behaviors, emotions and perception. Sex differences within the brain impact how we view ourselves, how we think about others and how we experience pain. These differences yield different neurological trajectories. Differences in these trajectories predispose many men to developing a susceptibility to and compulsions toward pornography. It starts playing out at the genetic level and continues throughout development.

GENETIC/CHROMOSOMAL SEX

The fact that there are biological differences between the sexes has long been recognized at the physical (that is external phenotypic) level, but we all started out as two halves. Before you were one being there were two cells; one cell made by your mother and one by your father. Since the time of conception when they joined together, every cell that you have ever produced in your body (with the exception of your sperm or ovum) has a genetic code that carries what can be called your genetic (or chromosomal) sex. The genotype—XX for females and XY for males—for sex has been fairly well understood for many decades. The presence of the pair of genes that influence the development of reproductive organs is one of the easier ways to identify the sex of an organism. These sex chromosomes express themselves differently because of either the presence of a single or double copy of a gene. Our many genetic differences affect our health, our bodies, our minds, our spiritual journey and our role in society (Arnold, 2004, pp. 701-8).

In species that have this small sperm and large ovum reproductive system, females will be very selective about the males that they choose to mate with. Because of the enormous amount of energy invested in producing the ovum, carrying the developing offspring and raising the newborn, a female must be very careful whom she mates with. A male, on the other hand, is able to produce a large number of sperm and is able to impregnate multiple females. It is because of this that many have argued that males are predisposed to seeking out as many sexual encounters as possible. This promiscuous approach is inherent in the reproductive system.

The desire for something new and different and the drive to constantly be seeking out multiple partners is driven not by a gene, but by the organ which governs their motivational systems (their brain) to do so. It is actually quite difficult to become a male. Many biologists say that nature's default is female; that all things being equal, an organism would much rather become a female than the male. This "fight to be male" begins with the race to become the first spermatozoa to reach the ovum. I once heard a pastor say, "Everyone in life is a winner because you were once a sperm that won the race to the ovum." I didn't have the heart to tell him that if he followed this line of reproductive reasoning, it only meant that genetically half of everyone is a "winner." The other half was waiting around and hoping not to be discarded.

The genetic heritage that a sperm cell gets from its father (who is XY) will be the determining factor in the sex of the child. This is referred to as *genetic* or *chromosomal* sex. There is a 50/50 chance that a sperm with a Y chromosome will reach the ovum and be the one that fuses with it to form the zygote. But the process of becoming male is not over yet. Once the Y chromosome contributed by the father fuses with the zygote, a specific set of genes in this new organism must be triggered, a process known as gene expression, in order for the next stage of becoming male to occur. The next step beyond genetic sex lies in the tissue that made the genetic half-complement sperm and egg cells that started it all: the gonads.

GONADAL SEX

Just because someone has a male genetic sex (XY) does not mean that they will automatically develop testes or the rest of their body will develop the full complement of male reproductive equipment. Located on the Y chromosome donated by the father is a gene known as the SRY gene. As the embryo is forming, this SRY gene turns on and produces a protein known as the SRY protein. This protein acts as the biological factor that causes the mass of tissue to become the reproductive organs that the child will possess. This tissue is referred to as gonadal tissue and develops into either the testes or ovaries. If this testis-determining factor produced by the SRY gene is not present during the early developmental stages of the child, the gonadal tissue does not become testes; it will develop into the ovaries. These gonads will develop into ovaries unless instructed otherwise, hence the thinking that female is nature's "default."

This is another level of sexuality known as *gonadal* sex. The gonadal sex will determine what type of cells the organism will produce in adulthood—sperm or ovum. The gonads produce the gametes that contain their half of the genetic material they will contribute to their offspring. In gonadal males the testes produce a number of substances, but special attention is given to testosterone. And while every cell in the body has the genetic code for being male, testosterone becomes the primary player for influencing the development of other parts of the body. The presence of testosterone during the first trimester and later at puberty has a profound impact on what kind of adult this person will grow up into. But even here in the womb, the embryo is not in a vacuum. The hormones that the mother produces or the things she ingests can also impact the development of the child (i.e., fetal

alcohol syndrome, DES [diethylstilbesterol] and other teratogens).
Where a person ends up as an adult is a complex web that begins at
conception, continues during intrauterine environment, and is influenced by their experiences as a child, during adolescence and then as
an adult.

The influence of testosterone in the embryo and fetus is not restricted to the reproductive organs; it affects everything else as
well. As testosterone courses throughout the developing child it affects muscle tissue, bones, lungs, the heart and numerous other sets
of tissue contributing to the biological differences between males
and females.

INTERNAL SEX

Between six and eight weeks after conception, before the embryo
becomes a fetus, the gonads have become either testes or ovaries and
the embryo's reproductive organs are preparing to be either male or
female. It has produced two sets of tissues: a female set known as
the Mullerian system and the male set known as the Wolfian system. As a general rule, the female system will be formed and continue to develop unless it is stopped. In a female, the Wolfian system
is present in the embryonic stage, but with the absence of testosterone it quickly disappears while the Mullerian system chugs along. In
males, however, the development of the Wolfian system results in
the internal male sexual organs such as the seminal vesicles and
prostate.

In the male, after the gonads have become testes two things have to
occur. The first is that the Mullerian system has to be stopped. The
embryo develops in the female mode by default, so the development of
the Mullerian system is stopped by the secretion of a hormone produced by the testes (called Mullerian inhibiting substance, MIS).
While this is occurring, the second step of saving the Wolfian system
begins. While MIS is shutting down the Mullerian system, the testes'
production of testosterone stimulates the Wolfian system and facili-
tates its development. Without testosterone the Wolfian system would

regress and disappear as it does in genetic and gonadal females. The development of the internal reproductive organs is what is referred to as the *internal* (or sometimes *internal phenotypic*) sex. The development of those internal tissues impacts the ability of that child to reproduce in adulthood.

But there is more to reproduction than what is inside of the organism, than the gonads that produce sperm or ovum, vas deferens or fallopian tubes, a prostate or a uterus. When a child is born, the first indicator of what sex they are is the external sex organs: the genitals.

GENITAL SEX

As testosterone and MIS set into motion the events to stop the female internal organs and to stimulate the male organs, the layers of tissue that will become the external genitalia are not produced in duplicate. There is only one set of tissue on the surface of the fetus, but again the presence of testosterone in the system is critical. While testosterone does not directly cause the genital tissue to become male, it does so indirectly. The breaking down of testosterone by the enzyme 5-alpha reductase leads to the production of dihydrotestosterone (DHT). DHT, known by many men as being involved in male pattern baldness, stimulates the developing genitals to become the penis and scrotum. Normally the external sex organs are used as an indicator (at either the time of birth or on the ultrasound) used to label someone male or female. This *genital* (or *external phenotypic*) sex is what many would say is the easiest way to determine if someone is a man or a woman, a boy or a girl. But because the gonads are cranking out testosterone, it goes to other tissue and organs as well.

BRAIN SEX

The different (and sometimes sexually dimorphic) brain regions are the result of a complex mix of genes, prenatal hormone levels and neurological/hormonal responses to life events. During fetal development the testosterone that is produced by the testes in males is sent throughout the developing child. These hormones affect the mother as well as the developing embryo. A good portion of this testosterone that is produced by the growing embryo finds its way into the developing brain. Sex hormones like estrogen and progesterone that are found in developing females do not pass into the brain. In females, the gonadal hormone estrogen does not pass into the brain because of a protein that latches onto it. This protein, called alpha-fetoprotein, is responsible for preventing estrogen from entering the brain. And why is it important that alpha-fetoprotein binds to estrogen and stops it from entering the brain? It is actually estrogen that makes a brain male.

Testosterone freely passes into the brain and then, through a process known as aromatization, it is converted into estrogen. This begins the process of tweaking how the brain lays down its neural circuits. This is what makes it a "male" brain, at least as far as sexual orientation goes. The regions of the brain that appear to be masculinized during early development are related more to wiring the brain so that it will be "turned on" by female cues when it is sexually mature.

This research is of interest for those who are examining the issue of homosexuality (Rahman, 2005, p. 1057). This masculinization of the male brain can be thought of as a *neurological sex* and has become an area of increased interest over the past few decades. But the issue extends beyond sexual orientation. There is gender identity (do I think of myself as a man or woman) as well. When discussing this with my students, I note that we often look at the external physical cues and behavior as indicators of personhood. From the outside my students would say that I am a heterosexual male, having male genitalia and opposite-sex orientation toward women. If I were a transgendered lesbian—a woman trapped in a man's body (gender identity) with a sexual orientation toward females—would my behavior be any different than a heterosexual man's? Mental gymnastics notwithstanding, there is a clear difference in the two. How the brain thinks of itself as a sexual creature and what cues arouse it are just two tiles in the neurological sexual mosaic that is being formed.

With the advent of brain imaging technologies, researchers have begun to explore the ways that the brains of men and women differ in their morphology, organization, connectivity and functionality. Throughout development, the brain is being rewired and constantly interacting with how it has internally processed information and understands itself and how it adapts to the incoming information from the world around it. Here we see how the social and religious systems can begin the backflow into the brain and influence how we think of our gender identity and the gender roles that we are assigned. The brain is plastic enough that gender roles may be socially influenced, but each person is restricted by the neurological boundaries that hormones and previous experience have set. For example, many exclusively heterosexual men resist the thought of engaging in a homosexual act, yet they find lesbian pornography arousing. The flexibility of what they find visually stimulating is restricted to female cues and not to the abstract concept of homosexuality.

FROM GENES TO THOUGHTS AND BEHAVIOR

As genes direct the gonads, and as gonadal hormones direct the brain in different ways at different times, our consciousness emerges from the brain. The brain is the organ where we think about and determine how to act on the world. But the story doesn't end here. The brain is dynamic and develops a hormonal mosaic of neural connections. Hormonal changes during puberty restructure the developing brain. Hormones other than testosterone (like stress hormones and adrenaline) change it throughout life. As the world acts on us, it changes our brains. As our brains change, our thoughts, behaviors and emotions are modified. The things that we see, habits we form and thoughts we think can alter the release of these hormones as well.

Testosterone organizes the male brain early in the womb and again during puberty. But testosterone does not disappear between these critical periods or after puberty. The ongoing production of testosterone has stimulating effects on the very organs it influenced during critical organizational periods of development. The flood of testosterone in the womb and during puberty creates a brain that is a sexual mosaic—different brain regions are hardwired for sexual arousal while other regions are left to be programmed by experience. The way that many males' brains have been hardwired and the software that they have been operating on leave them at risk for pornography addiction and problems with sexual compulsions.

REFERENCES

Arnold, A. P. 2004. Sex chromosomes and brain gender. *Nature Reviews Neuroscience* 5, no. 9 (Sept): 701-8.

Barth, K. 1977. *Church dogmatics*. G. W. Bromiley, T. F. Torrance and G. T. Thomson, trans. Edinburgh: T & T Clark.

Berenbaum, Sheri A., Krishna Korman and Catherine Leveroni. 1995. Early hormones and sex differences in cognitive abilities. *Learning and Individual Differences* 7, no. 4: 303-21.

Brown, W. S., N. C. Murphy and H. N. Malony. 1998. *Whatever happened to the soul?: Scientific and theological portraits of human nature*. Minneapolis: Fortress Press.

Chivers, Meredith L., and J. M. Bailey. 2005. A sex difference in features that elicit genital response. *Biological Psychology* 70, no. 2 (10): 115-20.

Einstein, Gillian, ed. 2007. *Sex and the brain: A reader*. Cambridge, MA: MIT Press.

Gregersen, N. H., W. B. Drees and U. Görman. 2000. *The human person in science and theology*. Edinburgh: T & T Clark; Grand Rapids, MI: Eerdmans.

Hoekema, A. A. 1986. *Created in God's image*. Carlisle, UK: Paternoster.

Jeeves, M. A. 2004. *From cells to souls and beyond: Changing portraits of human nature*. Grand Rapids, MI: Eerdmans.

Lewis, C. S. 1977. *The weight of glory*. Greensboro, NC: Unicorn Press.

Mealey, L. 2000. *Sex differences: Development and evolutionary strategies*. San Diego, CA: Academic Press.

Rahman, Qazi,. 2005. *The neurodevelopment of human sexual orientation*. New York: Pergamon.

6

Masculinity

ALL HUMAN BEINGS, MEN AND WOMEN, are created in the image of God. We are created for the purpose of knowing, loving and worshiping God and to live out our unique calling in this world. As followers of Christ, we are to conform to the image of Christ. How this manifests itself will be similar in some ways (we are all called to cultivate the fruit of the Spirit, Gal 5:22-25) and different in other ways depending on our embodiment (male or female), differences in personality and unique personal experiences. This does not mean that one form of embodiment, personality or experience is preferred. Nor should what is excellent in one be used to abuse and denigrate its absence in another person. Differences that may be more practical or efficient under some circumstances should not be used to devalue another. Because we are finite, we cannot be all things in all places at all times. Only together with other human beings do we transcend our individual embodied nature and more completely image God.

So what does it mean to be a man? How should we think about masculinity? Can the church share a vision of masculinity that is better than the one offered by the world? This vision must acknowledge and celebrate the embodied nature of the male while providing space for women. But men today often feel as if the church has become feminized and has no place for them. Without space for their longing for sanctification in the world, and without space for the expression of their male nature in the church, many men have started losing hope.

How do we get from male to masculine? How do we get from fe-

male to feminine? Can they both be valued and viewed as comple-
mentary? Can one be elevated without the denigration of the other?
Are there particular times in life where one must step to the front and
the other remains in place? Masculinity is not a singular thing. It has
many different dimensions that are restricted by the limitations of our
embodied biological and neurological wiring.

SEX AND GENDER

Understanding the biological process of male development of a male
sheds some light on the complexities behind the formation of masculine ideology. It is important to distinguish sex (a matter of biology)
from gender (masculinity, femininity) because the two are often used
interchangeably. A person's sex is best understood as referring to the
biological or physical characteristics of an individual's reproductive
organs. The terms *male* and *female* are best reserved for discussions
about sex. Gender, on the other hand, refers to the psychological, social, cultural and spiritual characteristics that have been associated
with the sex categories of male and female. Discussions about gender
use the terms *men* and *women*, or when dealing with psychological,
social, cultural or spiritual terminology, *masculine* and *feminine*.
Where sex is tied to reproductive physiology, gender is a cultural construct (McMinn, 2004).

Gender roles are behaviors that individuals engage in that are in
line with the socially constructed norms of masculinity and femininity attached to biological sex. Books like *Men Are from Mars, Women
Are from Venus* capitalize on the obvious physiological differences
and minimize our shared experience. It is important to understand
that there are significant differences between men and women that
are rooted our wiring, our neurological and physiological makeup.
Men and women image God both independently and together in distinct ways influenced by God's intentional design of their physical
bodies.

There should be no exclusive valuing of masculinity and the demeaning of femininity. Logic, abstract thinking and the concrete na-

ture with which many men interact with creation is not inherently superior to an intuitive, social and relational form found in the feminine. In many ways it is difficult to tap dance around the reality that Scripture sometimes refers to relationships as hierarchical and at other times as more egalitarian. In truth both of these dimensions are important, and at times the hierarchical nature between men and women must be exercised. When a situation calls for masculine attributes, they should be employed. When a situation calls for feminine attributes, they should be employed. At other times the egalitarian nature is to be preferred; the combination of masculine and feminine are to be employed together.

MASCULINITY

The past three decades the topic of masculinity has attracted a significant amount of academic investigation. It was a time when a "crisis in masculinity" developed (Payne, 1985; Van Leeuwen, 1990). Many men have shared with me that they feel bombarded by cultural accusations that they are hormone-driven, hedonistic, emotionless, violent, arrogant, promiscuous, idiotic, competitive oafs. Whether it is a cable television show like *MANswers*, beer commercials during baseball games, office memos about sexual harassment or the latest pseudo-scientific advice from "sexperts," men are told that they are the source of the majority of the world's problems.

Men also say that another message is that in order to become more human, they must become more feminine—sensitive, altruistic, faithful, intelligent and inclusive. Men are not encouraged to explore their emotions, nor are their emotions respected at the same level as a woman's. They are taught to respect a woman's emotions but are told that their own emotions are a sign of weakness.

Emotions are not, however, inherently feminine. Nor are they by nature manipulative. Emotions are human, not feminine. Tears are not always the "weapons of the weak." They can be the manifestation of pain, joy, relief, healing and forgiveness, not a sign of weakness. Weakness is a human trait, not a feminine trait.

Young girls physically develop more rapidly than boys, have a clear signal of their reproductive maturity (the onset of menstruation) and are often encouraged in their female embodiment. Boys (and men) are often told that women are superior emotional and linguistic beings. The confusion about what men are supposed to be (traditional or renaissance men), the lack of clarity with respect to how they should behave, and the absence of fathers and mentors to guide them is a recipe for dysfunctional masculinity.

LEARNING MASCULINITY

Masculinity is sensitive to religious and cultural ideologies, but these ideologies cannot deny the biological realities of the male nature. These ideologies, though, have their impact on the organ of mental life, the brain. The brain is flexible in how it adapts and responds to culture and society, able to store beliefs and wisdom within its synaptic wiring. These beliefs can change the way that it functions, limiting or expanding the cognitive, emotional and physiological ways that we respond to our environment. Masculinity emerges out of our embodied, biological nature and is informed and influenced by these beliefs. It is here in the brain where the culture nudges our embodiment and directs our actions, thoughts and beliefs. The brain of a boy is wired according to the male hormones that influenced its development, but it is not so hardwired that religious teaching and cultural forces cannot nudge it to fine tune its circuitry. These circuits are the embodied routes through which thoughts, emotions, desires and actions flow.

The masculine ideology is defined as an "endorsement and internalization of cultural belief systems about masculinity and male gender, rooted in the structural relationships between the two sexes" (Pleck, Sonenstein and Ku, 1993). As young boys grow they begin the process of developing this ideology. They detect both the cultural norms and expectations that surround what it means to be a man. They want to figure out what it means to be a man. Unfortunately social, cognitive, emotional and behavioral aspects of human nature are described as masculine or feminine and treated as if they are dichotomies (much like reproductive sex) rather than tendencies or predispositions influenced by hormonal effects on neurological development.

In the United States a considerable amount of research has looked at what exactly it means to be male. Two models of what are considered to be traditional masculinity are Brannon's blueprint for manhood and O'Neil's masculinity mystique model. Brannon's model describes four guidelines for men in the United States (Pleck, Sonenstein and Ku, 1993, pp. 85-110). These guidelines include (1) avoiding the appearance of being feminine, (2) attaining a high level of status and respect, (3) being invulnerable, and (4) seeking out adventure and opportunities to dominate (through use of force/violence). O'Neal's model focuses less on principles to guide men through life and more on norms to achieve. Men are to be (1) independence- and achievement-oriented, instrumental in their use of their time and resources; (2) dominant their interactions with others, avoiding relational styles which seem feminine or might infer homosexuality; and (3) rational, restricting and/or suppressing one's emotionality.

In these two models the masculine has social principles and norms that must be adhered to. As a boy becomes a "man," he internalizes these beliefs that encourage emotional disconnection, social investment and status seeking, and demeaning of feminine character traits. Women are viewed as weaker. When these norms or principles are absent or not held by a man, that man is viewed with contempt. He is unfit to stand with the company of "real men."

While most of the psychological research focuses on white middle-class men, there is now an increasing focus on masculinity in other cultural contexts. Marital status, race, social class, religion, ethnicity, intellectual ability, career, age and other factors all intersect with masculinity. This contributes to the difficulty that many boys and men have in learning what it means to be a man. Sometimes men must choose between competing norms of masculinity. Being an African American man, an Asian American man or a Mexican American man is different from being a white middle-class man. A married man and a bachelor have different norms. A father in his twenties feels the burden differently than a father in his forties.

The dominant conception of masculinity in American culture can be summarized like this: Men are assumed to be naturally competitive and aggressive, and being a "real man" is therefore marked by the struggle for control, conquest and domination. A man looks at the world, sees what he wants and takes it. This can be described as the "king of the hill" mentality. Unfortunately in this framework, there can be only one king. All others are destined for failure or a never-ending cycle of competition, violence, victory, vigilance, challenge and defeat. (Jensen, 2007).

As the father of a son, I have become acutely aware of how my life impacts the young man that I am raising. Each day as I go to work, love his mother, care for the house, coach soccer and wrestle with him, I model for him what he will use to determine appropriate and inappropriate behavior. I communicate to him through my words and actions how he is to treat his sisters, his mother and his friends. Just by living with me he begins to catch my understanding of what it is to be a man and use it to form his own understanding. He will watch how I treat his mother, whether it be with affection and honor or disdain and disrespect. He will see how I look at other women, with a steady glance or with a lecherous leer. He will notice the things I watch and entertain myself with, the books and magazines I read, the jokes I laugh at, the way I talk about people and the way I talk about sex. All of this is how a father models for his son not only what it means to be a man but how a man interacts with the women in his world. I can either be unintentional about this process, or I can be aware of it, harnessing myself, not only for my own sake but for his.

In the book *The Transformation of a Man's Heart*, John D. Pierce writes,

> Apart from the rejection of God, there are two significant rejections that can stunt a man's emotional, social and sexual growth. One is for a man's pursuit to be rebuffed by a woman. The sec-

ond is to be deemed unworthy to stand in the company of other men. (Smith, 2006, p. 132)

To be isolated from the community of men to which a man biologically belongs and to be considered inadequate in their company is a severe wound. It says that even the physical body is unable to hide the deficiency that is an even deeper part of what makes them who they are; they believe that underneath it all they are unworthy of the body that has been given to them.

Possessing a personality trait or acting in such a way that is considered feminine can lead many men to feel their masculinity is in question. Physical intimacy with other men is avoided at all costs and feeds homophobia and fear of being viewed as feminine. This puts them in a place of great concern, conflict and anxiety because men need to feel counted as equals among other men. It carries with it a form of male superiority.

There is a double standard of masculinity where the "traditional" role (strong, stoic, commanding) and the "renaissance man" (empathic, sensitive, egalitarian) collide. Mothers soothe and heal, fathers energize and challenge. Fathers cannot, and should not, be a male mother. They are crucial in the caring of both boys and girls. Fathers (and other male mentors) provide the model boys look to in order to understand their future. Fathers teach the skills necessary to flourish in a challenging world. One of the most important tools is emotional mastery. Emotional mastery is important because it teaches boys how to regulate and control their feelings. As a father pushes and challenges, he offers an opportunity for his son to experience these human emotions in a safe place. The son learns to name them as his father explains how to direct them appropriately, how to recognize that they are spiraling out of control and what to do to prevent them from doing so.

If a father does not have emotional mastery, then he cannot pass it along to his son. In the traditional model of masculinity, however, emotional mastery often masquerades as emotional repression or emotional inability. There should be little surprise at the result. As men grow up without these tools, their sexual drives and emotions become fueled by pornography. Regularly fueled sexual tension and emotion by pornography results in patterns of acting out that can be traumatic and disastrous.

Much of what is understood about historical gender roles is categorical. Men and women have been separated as a result of reproductive biology (external phenotype) and rigidly dictated social duties and responsibilities. There are hunters and gatherers, breadwinners and stay-at-home moms, providers and nurturers, chivalrous knights and damsels in distress. Unfortunately some aspects of these roles devolved into caricatures of male chauvinist pigs and submissive emotional women. These caricatures are still present and even celebrated in many corners of our culture (including Christianity), but they have been challenged in recent years. Because of the many abuses of traditional roles, with women usually on the receiving end of those abuses, the trend has been to deemphasize differences between the sexes. Thoughtful reflection by those who recognized the need to honor the image of God in women was combined with a political correctness that sought to punish men for years of patriarchic abuses. In doing so, the goal was to make men and women equal in every way.

This shifted society from a place where the masculine was celebrated and the feminine demeaned to one where the feminine was celebrated and the masculine demeaned. The intentions of honoring the dignity of both men and women resulted in something quite the contrary. Rather than elevate the feminine and celebrate it equally with the masculine, men were demeaned and androgyny was celebrated. This move toward a gender neutral perspective had men getting in touch with their feminine side and women getting in touch with their masculine side. In many ways this yielded positive steps— men free to express their emotionality, women freed to use all of their gifts. But the cultural shift has resulted in many negative consequences as well. The idealization of androgyny leads to the belief that everything is possible for everyone regardless of one's sex. It denies the biological reality that men and women are different and that our brains are uniquely wired as a part of our sexual development. Forced into believing that they are capable and obligated to have it all, women are finding that it doesn't work that way.

As women try to be more masculine, they become more depressed and stressed, frustrated by the unmet expectations and hollow promises of fulfillment if they are simply masculine. At the same time, men are told to be more feminine yet are forced into the culturally ostracized macho caricature. Men become less engaged and more passive, dispirited by the impossibility of it all. Feeling that nothing they do really matters or that it is too hard to do it all, too many men abandon their wives and children and seek only the passing fancies of the moment.

> Women had to overcome oppression, but men's difficulties are with isolation. The enemies, the prisons from which men must escape, are: loneliness, compulsive competition, and lifelong emotional timidity. Men's enemies are often on the inside—in the walls we put up around our own hearts. (Biddulph, 1994, p. 4)

But it is important not to confuse clear-minded thinking that honors the feminine with anti-masculine vitriol. Man-hating does no benefit to femininity, nor does misogyny to masculinity. Having sat through my share of conversations with an all-male group where the consensus was "all women are evil" and having eavesdropped on the female counterpart that "all men are evil," I find both to be exaggerations of the greatest fears that the sexes have of each other. Granted, the majority of these conversations occur either during critical developmental times (junior high through college when sexual/dating/ relationship tensions run high) or as a result of shared experience (divorce recovery groups). The function of these groups is to circle the wagons and help bring the wounded party back to a place of emotional and psychological health. After socially sanctioned group behaviors to deal with the initial pain (such as eating ice cream or going to a strip club) and writing in same-sex groups to protect the wounded party, the pain subsides and reason usually prevails.

Not all men are evil, nor are all women evil. All people do bad, mean, selfish, careless things. Most people are just unaware of how easily and innocently we can wound the other sex. To follow the path of sanctification when driven by your sexual nature requires a discerning spirit. This spirit of discernment is needed to know what way is best to discipline your response so that you are driven to the heart of God rather than into the consumption of his image in other people.

Being male has its "privileges," but these are often mixed with burdens. In some cases the expectations and privileges of being a man lead them along paths where they feel compelled to do things that are inherently harmful to themselves and others. Much of the feminist critique of men is rooted in the belief that men are fundamentally creatures who exercise power over women. This power is used to manipulate women for the selfish desires and needs. If this is the case, then pornography is perhaps the easiest way to objectify, degrade, subjugate and consume women.

But this is not the entire story. It would be dishonest to say that women do not have any power over men. Indeed the free offering of a woman's love and respect to a man meets his deepest needs to be loved and accepted. This does not mean that men always act in a lovable or respectable manner; in most cases we don't, but that is because we are all imperfect and (ideally) moving toward greater sanctification. Sanctification in this world does not happen immediately, as if the Holy Spirit waves a magic wand over us and, poof, we are perfect. But the same is true for women. One of the underlying messages that many men hear in the feminist critique is that to be male is inherently evil and that attempts to become a better person will be difficult at best because of our biological makeup, as if the depravity of humanity were restricted to men alone. The doctrine of depravity is true for all human beings, men and women.

Christian men especially feel betrayed by this because they do recognize ways that a feminist critique of masculinity is dead on. They respond positively to the need for men to find ways that allow their maleness to be expressed in godly, loving ways. But these ways are not godly because they are feminine. They are godly because they are rooted in the image of God that is placed in every person.

A BIBLICAL UNDERSTANDING

Within Christianity, the masculine image of God is often defined in these terms of control, power and dominion. Much of the Christian faith, though, requires that men recognize their limitations and depend on God. We accept salvation through his son and sanctification by the power of the Holy Spirit. It is a faith where the last shall be first (Mk 10:31), marked by a life of service to others. If the culture labels these attitudes as feminine, how can Christianity be masculine?

American culture is saturated with stereotypes of macho posturing, sexual promiscuity, aggression and competitive one-upmanship. At times they are celebrated and at other times they are denigrated. Confused about their purpose and identity, men spiral into doubt about their own value and worth. Consider the definition offered by John Piper: "At the heart of mature masculinity is a sense of benevolent responsibility to lead, provide for and protect women in ways appropriate to a man's differing relationships" (Piper and Grudem, 2006, p. 35). It is a definition that emphasizes leading, providing for and protecting women. But it offers no insight on how men relate to one another. Depending on your reading of this definition, it either smacks of male chauvinism or places greater value on women's needs. No doubt well intentioned, it offers little guidance for men who are already confused, wounded and lost about their masculinity.

In an article titled "The Top 10 Things Promise Keepers Has Learned About Men," Tom Fortson (2006) wrote that men who attended Promise Keepers gatherings struggled with a number of issues. They were:

1. Friendlessness. They had few friends that knew them well.

2. Emotional isolation. They had no outlet or tools to deal with their

emotional needs. This was particularly true of pastors and church
leaders who felt an even greater sense of isolation.

3. Confusion about masculinity. They were unsure of a right way to
understand their male nature.

4. Success-driven. There was a constant need to be successful in all
aspects of life; they felt they would always be evaluated on their
performance.

5. Spiritually searching. There were spiritual needs that had been unmet. In many cases, these men had moved to alternative faith communities outside the institutional church.

We know that Jesus was a male and that he had presumably been
taken to the temple to be circumcised, but we know precious little
about his sexuality otherwise. Scripture and church tradition indicate
that his life was celibate and the Gospel accounts contain little instruction in the area of sexuality. When Jesus does address it, he
stresses sexual fidelity in the marital relationship.

Many Christian men are concerned that while the face of Christianity is changing as a result of political correctness and liberal feminist theology (many see the terms "liberal" and "feminist" as being
inseparable), they are somehow losing the heart and soul of their faith.
If this feminized version of Christianity is really at the heart of the
faith, then they would rather look elsewhere.

At times we like to think of Jesus as Rambo. We see in Scripture
that Jesus comes with a sword and that he defeats the armies of Satan
(very warlike, isn't it?). This was perhaps the biggest problem with the
Jews of Jesus' time. They were expecting a Rambo Jesus. Okay, maybe
not a Rambo Jesus, but at least a King David Jesus. King David was a
military leader that went out and defeated the enemies of Israel. He
also had some other issues, like killing the husband of a woman he
slept with, deceiving his people and poor parenting skills.

The wimpy, androgynous Jesus that meekly dotes on the weak and
allows himself to be killed is not exactly the archetypal male. But nei-

ther do we seek a Rambo Jesus. He does not go out and kick butt. Rather than blame the so-called "liberal feminist theologians" or the feminist movement for the demasculinization of today's men, perhaps we should step back and look at some other cultural factors.

The culture has lied to both men and women and fed us all stereotypes about brutish men, incapable of tenderness and of winsome women full of sensitivity and empathy. I have certainly met some stereotypic, brutish men who have been hindered in their ability to feel anything for another human being, and I have met some stereotypic women who feel deeply for others and connect with people in their places of brokenness. But I have also met some stereotype-smashing women who are brutish, and I have met some stereotype-smashing men who have displayed tender care for other human beings.

As created beings we are limited in how we hold the many aspects of the character of God given to us as bearers of his image. We are simply unable to be God and to hold all of these realities in tension. Only in the incarnation of Christ do we see the perfect union of strength and weakness, justice and mercy.

DIRECTING AND EMPOWERING MASCULINITY

The model of masculinity that has been passed down from our fathers and their fathers is untenable today. Much of that model is no longer relevant in the world we now live in. The models of masculinity that are offered in today's media are a hodgepodge of stupidity to genius, sensitivity to stoicism, violence to frailty, gluttony to discipline and nobility to depravity. So many confusing signals are being sent, but the vast majority of them depict men as Neanderthal boors that chase skirts, drink beer and watch sports. They either let the world pass them by or take it by the throat and force themselves upon it.

Masculinity should be understood as having a core to it that is the expression (on average) of God's image in ways that male embodiment enables. To contrast the masculine and feminine as always diametrically opposed misunderstands these expressions. Rather than address what "biblical" masculinity looks like, perhaps it is better to think of how the Bible directs the masculine nature. Is there something about being a new creation in Christ that requires that our masculinity changes?

As we explore core dimensions of the masculine journey toward sanctification, do not assume that women are unable to possess any of the following aspects. In many ways women also share in these very human needs, but they are more peripheral to core femininity. Also, do not assume that the opposite of any of the following traits must be core to femininity. In some cases, the opposite is sinful, not feminine. There is much to being human, and not all of it requires polar opposites that are forced results of our reproductive organs. Just as with masculinity, there is a core of femininity that is human first. Men may also share these needs, but these are more core to the process of sanctification to women.

Masculinity and femininity need not always be in tension with each other. This is often how our culture understands gender, and this sometimes creates unnecessary conflict. But if we understand how male and female, masculine and feminine, are together human, we can begin with human needs and embodiment then move to gender. Human nature need not be thought of as a dichotomy. Men and women have similar needs, yet their embodied nature may allow for their expression in different (but not antagonistic) ways. If we reconceptualize our thinking of masculinity as human first and then male, we need not compare or contrast it with femininity or female nature.

What is unfortunate is that masculinity is often times described as a singular thing. The lie of the singularity of masculinity is that there is an ideal man that we should aspire to be. This ideal can be thought of as a cultural icon such as John Wayne, Clint Eastwood or Arnold Schwarzenegger. The lie that is foisted upon men both young and old is that if we are like them, we have arrived. We would be fully masculine and reap all of the benefits that go along with it, such as the respect and admiration of our male peers and the desire of women. But masculinity does not have a single model of expression. There are multiple ways of being masculine.

THE MASCULINE VOICE AFFIRMS

The voice of the masculine speaks to affirm. All children are carried and primarily nourished by the mother. Daughters and sons first know their mother as she carries them, delivers them into the world and then is their primary source of nourishment. In many ways the child moves from becoming an extension of the mother to their own person. All children, both boys and girls, develop their own sense of identity as they separate from their mother. For boys, this process is fairly straightforward. What makes them different from their mothers is fairly easy to see: their bodies.

Both young boys and young girls need to hear from both the feminine and the masculine voice. These voices can be spoken by both mothers and fathers. A father is not incapable of nurturing because he is a man, neither is a mother incapable of affirming because she is a woman. But the masculine voice alone speaking both affirmation and nurture is not enough. The feminine voice speaking both nurture and affirmation is not enough either.

Does this mean that a child who grows up in a house where one of their parents is not present is doomed to a life of truncated emotional, psychological and spiritual development? Not if there is a male presence other than the father that is able to come in and act as a surrogate for those children. Boys and girls both need a masculine voice in their life that encourages, affirms, challenges, enables and stretches them. In an ideal set of circumstances both mother and father are present in the raising of a child. Both the masculine and the feminine speak to nurture, protect and grow, albeit in different ways.

There is something special about the affirming voice of the masculine father. This voice of affirmation is not just needed for young men, but also for young women. While it may be true that "only a father can tell a boy when he is a man" (and worthy to stand among his peers), it is also true that the father's affirmation of a daughter's worth speaks into her being in a way that others do not.

The voice of affirmation does not affirm based on performance. Many men fall into the trap of affirming their children only when the child meets the behavioral criteria for acceptance. Hitting a home run, scoring a goal, getting straight As, winning an award or landing a great job may be the only times children hear their father say, "Well done." Indeed, mothers bear an unfair burden of the blame when fathers don't speak as the affirming voice into their children's lives. The mother, who is supposed to be the child's primary source of nurture, is forced to challenge and discipline.

When the one whom we come from says that we are not good, it runs counter to what she should know to be true: that she is good. If a mother believes herself to not be good, then what comes from her (particularly her children) are also not good. But if a mother believes herself to be good (and why shouldn't she?) would she not then believe that what comes from her is good as well? This is why the affirming voice of the feminine does not carry the same weight that the affirming voice of the masculine does. It does not mean that the affirming voice of the feminine is entirely void. The voice of affirmation that comes from the feminine carries a different kind of weight. The masculine voice of affirmation spoken to a man lets him know that he is worthy to stand in the company of his peers; he is loved because of who he is. The masculine voice of affirmation spoken to a woman lets her know that she is loved because of who she is and that she is worthy of pursuit.

But when a boy realizes that he is other than his mother (his body is different and she acknowledges that he is different), who is it that tells him who he is, what he is to do, what he will become? His father. The father, the masculine voice, acts to inform, equip, instruct and model. In the absence of this voice, which at its best is loving, trustworthy and affirming, a boy is forced to look for whatever is available to discover who he is. He may look to his mother for instruction, and she rightly has much to say on this matter, her guidance on how a man should relate comes from a female perspective. He may look to another male figure in his life; a grandfather, uncle, elder brother or the media.

The masculine voice is received as a voice that speaks unchanging truth. Just as we think of the Word of God being truth that is unchanging, so a man's words speak what he knows to be true. The Promise Keepers movement of the 1990s hit this nail on the head. When a man makes a promise, he is honor bound to keep it because his word is who he is. The degree to which a man keeps his word is the measure of his integrity and his honor. When the masculine voice affirms, it says, "It is good." It doesn't say, "It is okay now, but it might not be later." The affirming nature of God is evidenced in the first chapter of Genesis after the many acts of creation. God "saw that it was good" (Gen 1:4, 10, 12, 18, 21, 25, 31).

THE MASCULINE GROWS AS IT IS CHALLENGED

The masculine nature requires a task to be done, an obstacle to overcome, a cause to champion. Men love to compete, to acquire new skills, to adventure. Men grow as they are challenged. Men also need to know that they are progressing. Men need ways to measure their effectiveness. This is why so many young men love video games. They provide a sense of power and control of one's destiny. This need for power underlies the masculine need to be effectual. Video games allow a safe place for accomplishment, challenge and freedom to try new things while enjoying the creativity of others.

Consider the video game *Guitar Hero*. In *Guitar Hero,* players strum a guitar as they press colored buttons on the neck corresponding to colored notes scrolling down the screen. The game can be played solo, in a cooperative mode with another player or in a competitive mode pitting two players against each other. Players are given points for the correct fretting of notes, improvisational whammying of long notes (yes, the faux guitar has a tremolo bar—the more realistic and creative the better), and can advance levels to unlock hidden songs. It is like air guitar on steroids. It allows the player to not only pretend to be one of the ultimate male teenage archetypes of our age (the rock guitarist), but to advance and see how they compare to their peers.

Why bother actually learning how to play a real guitar (which is slightly more complex) and have your ability measured subjectively when you can get immediate feedback and rating through a video game? If playing guitar is not your thing, you can try out *Rock Band,* which offers the option of playing the bass guitar or drum and even has a microphone so that you can be the front man. Why go through the hassle of actually learning how to play music when you can pretend to? I don't offer many predictions, but I think it is only a matter of time before these video games are sexualized with the addition of groupies and the backstage rendezvous.

Rather than spend life adrift, constantly responding, the healthy masculine nature initiates. It creates. It faces challenges and grows as a result.

THE MASCULINE RESPONSE TO EVIL IS TO DEFEND

There are few better uses for the physical, emotional and spiritual power that men have then to defend that which is good, noble, pure and right. The stories that stir men's hearts often deal with war and aggression. The thought of oppression, slavery and the denigration of our loved ones lights a fire in men's hearts that drives them to sacrifice their lives. Movies like *300* and television shows like *Band of Brothers* appeal to the need that men have to use their strength to defend. This longing to sacrifice a man's life for something other than himself is good, but when corrupted, it becomes dominance and aggression. By exercising his power in a way to dominate, the masculine exerts his will to the damage of others.

In her book *My Brother's Keeper,* Mary Stewart Van Leeuwen (2002) frames masculinity as a product of our culture. It is "not something that just happens to us by reason of biology or socialization, though . . . these too are important." One of the more compelling theological premises that she offers can be related to the problems with impulse control. In her view, the image of God in men is related to the representative cultural mandate of *dominion* (Gen 1:28). In many men, this is corrupted and becomes *domination.* Men illegitimately exercise this aspect of the *imago Dei* by imposing themselves through their physical power. They do so on creation, on each other and on women. Often understood as core to the concept of masculinity, the caring control and dominion that mirrors God is warped and becomes a need to dominate, subject and rule over. But the heart of true masculinity is to defend.

CONCLUSION

Men and women have the same human needs because we are all human. We all think, feel, desire and seek purpose. We all communicate, love, work, play, wonder, socialize and look for meaning. None of the items listed above as part of the core of masculinity are exclusively male. Women also have a voice, need for purpose and growth.

Biblical, redeemed, true masculinity gives freely of its gifts, surrendering itself for the benefit of others, not just itself. It affirms, admonishes and brings peace and order. It does not condemn, dominate or bring chaos. As Christians, we reject the culture's corrupted understanding and celebration of biological and fallen masculinity. We reclaim a right understanding of our created masculinity and offer a vision of an embodied, redeemed man of God anchored in the incarnation of Christ.

This notion of differentiation, that aspects of our body become more specialized, fits with the biblical view that the image of God is reflected in two forms—male and female. Masculinity may be less hardwired in the brain than male sexual arousal and response, but the plastic, "soft" wired regions of the brain where beliefs about masculinity are maintained have a far-reaching effect in other areas of a man's life.

Our culture twists men's understanding of masculinity, trapping them and restricting them to an unhealthy and corrupt understanding of their sexuality. It limits the options they have to express their human and masculine nature. These factors contribute to pornography's ability to hijack a man's mental world and direct him toward thoughts and actions that lead him away from holiness. Our culture has taught men to deny one side of their humanity by calling it feminine and excluding it.

For the Christian, masculinity is best seen in the person of Jesus, who is fully God and fully man. His life, attitudes and behaviors are the best model for all men. In Jesus' humanity we see the perfect combination of the categories that many culturally define as masculine (strength, righteousness, rationality) and feminine (tenderness and compassion). These are what God desires within every human being, though men and women may be predisposed to express them differently.

REFERENCES

Biddulph, Steve. 1994. *Manhood: A book about setting men free.* Sydney: Finch Publishing.

Fortson, Tom. 2006. The top 10 things Promise Keepers has learned about men. *Christian Counseling Today* 14 (1), 36-39.

Jensen, Robert. 2007. *Getting off: Pornography and the end of masculinity.* Cambridge, MA: South End Press.

McMinn, Lisa G. 2004. *Sexuality and holy longing: Embracing intimacy in a broken world.* San Francisco: Jossey-Bass.

Payne, L. 1985. *Crisis in masculinity.* Wheaton, IL: Crossway Books.

Piper, John, and Wayne Grudem, eds. 2006. *Recovering biblical manhood and womanhood.* Wheaton, IL: Crossway Books.

Pleck, J. H., F. L. Sonenstein and L. C. Ku. 1993. Masculinity ideology and its correlates. *Gender issues in contemporary society:* 85–110.

Smith, Stephen W., ed. 2006. *The transformation of a man's heart.* Downers Grove, IL: InterVarsity Press.

Van Leeuwen, M. S. 1990. *Gender & grace: Love, work & parenting in a changing world.* Downers Grove, IL: InterVarsity Press.

Van Leeuwen, M. S. 2002. *My brother's keeper: What the social sciences do (and don't) tell us about masculinity.* Downers Grove, IL: InterVarsity Press.

7

The Male Need for Intimacy

"Our sexuality is a fundamental part of what it means to be human. How we understand it and experience it is integral as we discover who we are and it points us to our Creator. While it is fundamental to our being, our sexuality is not about sexual intercourse. Our sexuality is one of the sources of the restlessness in our lives. It drives us to search for intimacy where we can be fully known and where we can know another. It is in this place of intimacy where the experience of the ecstatic is sometimes met and we are able to transcend our physical limitations and understand in part the transcendent nature of God."

LISA McMINN, *SEXUALITY AND HOLY LONGING*

HUMAN BEINGS HAVE NEEDS FOR FOOD AND WATER. Without them we die; they are survival needs. But life is not just about surviving. We also have needs for protection, such as shelter and clothing, and we have needs for relationships. We rely on others to care for us as we grow; we form communities and have affiliations with others. A child needs the care of his parents when he is young. When he is older he forms friendships, looks for a mate, contributes to the community and cares for others. While each person may experience these needs differently, they are not essential for survival; you cannot die from loneliness, celibacy or failing to join a social club. Meeting these relational needs, however, is part of having a full life.

Table 7.1. Maslow's Hierarchy of Needs

Self-actualization needs
Need to live up to one's fullest
and unique potential

Esteem needs
Need for self-esteem, achievement,
competence and independence;
need for recognition and
respect from others

Belongingness and love needs
Need to love and be loved, to belong and be accepted;
need to avoid loneliness and alienation

Safety needs
Need to feel that the world is organized and predictable;
need to feel safe, secure and stable

Physiological needs
Need to satisfy hunger and thirst

Psychologist Abraham Maslow suggested that some needs have priority over others. Physiological needs related to surviving and subsistence like breathing, thirst and hunger must be met before higher needs like self-esteem, respect and self-actualization can be met. In Maslow's hierarchy we see that the relational needs like belonging, love and acceptance are superseded by the lower survival needs. Once these physiological needs are met, we are driven by sequentially higher needs. Being deprived of a need creates a state of tension. This state, called a drive, motivates us to satisfy the need. In the absence of food and water, we feel hungry and thirsty. In the absence of relationship and safety we feel lonely and vulnerable. We are pushed and pulled forward to reduce these drives. Needs push us into action, and the objects of their fulfillment (food, water, relationships, sexual intimacy/reproduction, clothing, a safe shelter) act as incentives, pulling us forward. Unlike God, we are not self-sufficient. To be human is to be created and finite. These drives fuel the growth, development and maturation of human beings.

Not surprisingly Scripture often describes God as the provider of our needs. The Lord is our hiding place, our shelter (Ps 27:5; 91:1). In the sacrament of communion, Jesus is offered as the bread of life (Mk 14:22-25). Jesus offers the water of life to the woman at the well (Jn 4:7-15). For every need that we experience in this world we see that God is the provider. Underneath it all our need for him is even more fundamental than our needs for food, drink, clothing, shelter and relationship. These needs are necessary parts of our created nature that help us pursue God. They are not just for our own pleasure, but point us toward the God who sustains us.

DRIVES AND SANCTIFICATION

A right understanding of our drives is found when we locate them as pointers to God rather than inconveniences of embodiment. Drives for food and water are the embodied manifestation of humanity's need for God's provision and sustenance. These drives are dynamic and are critical in the process of sanctification. Sanctification is the process by which we are made holy. It is the process by which we become what we are intended to be: fully mature, fulfilling our intended purpose. This process of sanctification extends into our relational needs and how human beings are made in the image of God.

Relational drives (including the sexual drive) propel us toward each other and toward God. In connecting with each other and knowing one another, we sample the transcendence of God. As we know and experience more of the other, we escape our finitude and understand the transcendence of God more clearly. We experience the intimate knowing that God longs for us to have for him, to know him as holy and good. Whether that transcendence is found in sexual union with a spouse or in the selfless giving of our time and affection to others, we can discover something outside of ourselves and experience the love, holiness and goodness of the Creator as we give selflessly to others.

Because we are embodied, we are to a certain extent alone. Just as we are finite and God is infinite, we are unique individuals whose nature is to be alone but long to not be alone. In the redemption of our broken sexuality on the path toward sanctification, we move toward the wholeness that fully occurs only when Christ returns or we are resurrected in the new heaven and earth. Communion with God and one another is the answer to the longing that our very nature craves. It can be found in friendships, the body of Christ, the expression of our sexuality and in many other ways. The mercy, grace and healing that can be found along the way both deepens our need for communion and our ability to have it (Balswick and Balswick, 1999).

Sanctification is the process by which we become what we are intended to be, fully mature and fulfilling our intended purpose (White, 2001). This process of sanctification extends into our sexuality. Whether someone is single or married, the process of sanctification can continue. The single person is able to become sanctified with respect to their sexuality in a way that is different than someone who is married and able to engage in sexual activity with a spouse. Both a husband and wife are able to become sanctified as they honor each other and their sexual relationship. The single person is able to experience God's provision in celibacy in a way that the married couple are unable to. In the same way the married couple is able to experience God's provision in a way that the single person is unable to. Regardless of one's marital status the continuing process of sanctification extends into each individual's sexuality.

Our sexual nature is an aspect of our created nature; it is a necessary part of us. It is not a warped part that must be fought against (Balswick and Balswick, 1999). It is a force that we must harness and direct to aid in the process of becoming holy. If we think of our sexual nature as fundamentally evil, as having only reproductive value or primarily for the experiencing of pleasure, we misunderstand the place of our sexual drives. The human sexual drive is a force of need, much like hunger and thirst. We have needs because we are finite. Our bodies use water and energy and so we must replenish them in order to survive. These needs are not an end in and of themselves but the means by which we become sanctified.

The sexual longings that we feel are part of our need for intimacy—to know and be known. Just as God is relational (as Father, Son and Holy Spirit), so the image of God is reflected in human relationships. Sexual intimacy is considered by many the highest form of intimacy two people may share with each other. But intimacy is more than just knowledge of details. True intimacy is found when there is an emotional connection between persons. Intimacy is found when goodness is spoken to each other. In Genesis 1 God does not just know creation, but knows it as *good*.

Men are driven to earn the respect of their coworkers or compete with their teammates. These drives are relational but are not *reproductive*. Most men would rather compete with other men than with women. The sex of the competitor is critical to them. But there are also drives between men that are related to reproduction. A son is driven to earn the respect of his father in a way that is different from how he relates to his mother. A father is driven to protect and care for his son in a way that is different from how he cares for his daughter. These relational drives between men, between father and son, teammates and coworkers are different from the relationships a man may have with a woman. The fabric of these relationships is informed by the common bonds they share as men. A man may have sexual drive toward his spouse, a drive to see his mother honored, or a drive to protect and nurture his daughter. These relational drives are rooted in his male nature and her female nature—they are rooted in their differences.

SEXUAL ENERGY

Every man experiences it. A woman enters the room, crosses the street or suddenly appears on the screen in front of him and it happens. He feels the energy coursing through his body. He is unable to see or think about anything other than her. The sight of her holds his gaze like a magnetic force and a fire within him is lit. He feels alive; he wants to know more of her.

Unfortunately, many men mistake this attraction as inherently erotic. They have not learned how to be affected by a woman's beauty or her presence without understanding it as erotic. They have trained themselves to interpret all such arousal and energy as only relating to intercourse (Ågmo, 2008, pp. 312-14). Their autonomic intelligence has only a handful of options to interpret arousal: be afraid of it, aggress against it or mate with it (Ariely and Loewenstein, 2006, p. 87). The problem with many men is that they need to open themselves up to understanding how to make sense of this arousal and use it in healthy ways. For the unmarried man it may be an opportunity to pursue her as a wife (if she is unmarried). For the married man, it can be a reminder of his first love, toward whom he can then direct this energy when he returns to his bride.

Sexual attraction is relational energy; it pushes us. It is rooted in the relational image of God. The tension we experience when the drive for intimacy kicks in propels us to seek communion with others. Human sexuality allows for the mystery, beauty, diversity and complexity of human life to be explored and for deepening bonds of intimacy to be formed. We have to move away from thinking that the sole purpose of our sexuality is intercourse.

When the need to be known is met regularly, the sexual drive is decreased. When it is not regularly satisfied, the force of it builds. As the drive increases, we become less able to make wise decisions about how we meet it. A starving man will eat anything that is put before him. An intimacy-neglected man will grasp at any available opportunity to know or be known. The need for intimacy will build without emotional connection, and he will look for this connection in unhealthy and unproductive places (such as pornography, strip clubs or prostitutes). These places and experiences do not truly meet the need for intimacy, so the drive will return quickly. It is only temporarily assuaged by these imposters. These emotional experiences are designed to have relational objects—real people—which anchor them.

The intimacy-starved man is analogous to someone who tries to meet his body's need for food by only eating chocolate. It may taste good, but it doesn't meet the true needs of the body. The body needs a complete diet, not just sugar. It needs vitamins and minerals. A diet of pure sugar makes the body obese, sluggish, underdeveloped and can lead to diabetes. The need for intimacy is like the need for a complete diet. It has many dimensions that are best satisfied through multiple means, not just the sugar of sexual relations.

Sexual development has social and spiritual implications that influence how a man responds psychologically to sexual stimuli. Men may be surprised to see how rooted in their biology they are, while at the same time marveling in the non-biological aspects of sexuality. The need for intimacy and relationality can manifest itself easily in romantic and sexual energy within a man. As he knows and is known by his mate, he experiences pleasure and transcendence in that union. This experience is stored in the wiring of his brain, binding him to his mate. This leads him to seek her out again when the need to know and be known reemerges.

The natural high that we get where we engage in sexual activity, especially the orgasm that a male experiences, exists for a purpose— to bind us to one another. Our capacity to experience these kinds of highs exists outside the realm of sexuality as well. Eating, drinking, athletics and even ecstatic religious experiences have an element of transcendence where we are able to momentarily escape our limitedness, our finiteness, and be in union with something outside of ourselves. We all long for intimacy and for the transcendence that comes when we experience it. Intimacy is the process by which we understand and grow toward our purpose in life: to be conformed to the image of Christ. It requires that we do as Christ did, to give of ourselves in acts of loving kindness and servant sacrifice for the benefit of others.

Understanding the person as an embodied, incarnate creation of God acknowledges our sexual nature and sees it not merely for the purpose of reproduction, but as an innate pointer toward our Creator. Our sexual longings drive us toward that place of intimacy with another human being. They offer a taste of the ecstasy that is found more perfectly when we are in communion with God. As our needs for food, water, clothing and shelter point us toward the deeper needs whereby God sustains, covers and protects us, our sexuality points us toward God as the one who meets our needs for intimacy and transcendence.

Just as the need for food and water may be sated after a meal or drink, so our needs for intimacy and transcendence can be met through our sexuality. Only God is unchanging. We will be forever in a state of change as we eat, digest and become hungry again. So our need for intimacy and transcendence builds, is satisfied and then slowly builds again as we are separated from our beloved. Because we are finite, we go through these cycles. These cycles can have an upward spiritual trajectory.

I remember one conversation with a man who thought I was naïve about male sexuality. He said, "Men are biologically driven to mate with as many women as possible. It's evolution. We can't help ourselves. It's what we are made to do."

"Really?" I asked.

"Yeah. We're made to spread our genes to as many different women as possible. We're programmed to look for new women to mate with."

"But what if you could find one woman who could be constantly changing? What if she was always different and could meet that need for novelty in a partner? Would that satisfy you?"

"You mean she wore sexy lingerie or dyed her hair?"

"No. I mean that as you got to know her better, you discovered dimensions of her that were so interesting that she became like a new woman."

"How's that?" he asked.

"What if you got to be promiscuous with your wife because your understanding of her was always changing? What if you discovered things about her that made her always new, always fresh? She could be a new woman for you to pursue each day."

"That woman doesn't exist."

"That woman does exist," I responded. "She's my wife. That's how I meet any 'evolutionary' need for promiscuity that I might have. I intentionally love her and discover new things to appreciate about her. She's not the same person I married years ago. In some ways she is the same, in some ways she's changed, and there are new things that I am discovering about her even now after more than a decade of being married. She is always different and exciting. Our relationship is like promiscuity within a monogamous relationship."

"You must have a pretty cool wife. My wife's not like that. But if you could bottle that, I'd buy it for her."

This man severely underestimated the complexity and beauty of his wife. He also failed to see the power that changing the way he thought about her might impact his desire for her. I have yet to meet a woman who thought that the notion of promiscuity in a monogamous marital relationship was unbiblical or unhealthy. I hear the appeal to evolution and the need for many partners from many men. But even when these attitudes are present, they can be captured and channeled in a loving relationship and propel both husband and wife toward sanctification.

TYPES OF INTIMACY

There is a form of intimacy that human beings were created to experience. It was an intimacy that was shared between God, Adam and Eve in the garden of Eden. In Genesis we see humanity before the Fall.

Both Adam and Eve are naked and unashamed. They are joined relationally with God and with each other. They are joined with each other sexually, with the fullest of pleasure. There is no hesitation, no self-doubt, no sense of incompleteness when they are with each other. This can be thought of as *perfect intimacy* (Schaumburg, 1992).

Unfortunately, after the Fall there is not only separation from God, but also between Adam and Eve. The perfect intimacy that they experienced with their Creator and with each other has been replaced with fear, shame and a desire to cover themselves. The intimacy that they experienced with each other is replaced by finger-pointing and blaming. This affects us all to this day. If we cannot have ongoing perfect intimacy, what forms of intimacy can we experience now?

It may be that in the future kingdom, perfect intimacy will again be realized and the moments of transcendence and healing in this life are signs of the kingdom to come. In our post-Fall state, human beings still bear the image of God in which we were created. But even in our fallen state, the Fall has not robbed us of hope for any form of intimacy. We are still relational, we are still sexual, and we still have a longing to know and to be known. The sexual intimacy shared with a spouse within a committed marriage where both are devoted to a life of obedience to God's will and submission to each other provides an opportunity to progress toward intimacy that is similar to that perfect intimacy. Self-doubt exists, but couples communicate relationally and sexually in ways that help them manage the realities of our post-Fall state.

We all face disappointments and have fears of exposure, abandonment, insufficiency and loss of control. Our sexual desires, which were part of our original design, echo the longing to be sexually known and open to each other. There is vulnerability and uncertainty in this form of intimacy, but as we bear the image of God rightly—loving each other according to his commands and directing our sexuality in accordance with Scripture—the intimacy that a man and a woman have builds toward perfect intimacy. This *maturing intimacy* bears the realities of our post-Fall condition, but is a sign of God's transforming power to overcome that condition.

Maturing intimacy is more than a romantic attraction or sexual chemistry. It is rooted in the agape love that we are to have for one another. It is marked by forgiveness, mercy, grace and perseverance. We have the emotional and spiritual drives to develop a relationship which meets our needs to know and to be known by another, but these needs find their fulfillment when they align with God's direction as revealed in Scripture. When those drives are properly directed, the result is truly beautiful to behold: a husband and wife who have devoted themselves to each other.

This form of maturing intimacy is what healthy men should experience. Perfect intimacy with one's spouse may be unrealistic in our current state, but the married man who is becoming sanctified has the opportunity to mature toward that perfect intimacy. It is important to note that this maturing intimacy is not restricted to husband-wife relationships, but the sexual form of intimacy (and remember, there are many forms of intimacy) is restricted to men and women within a marriage. A father should have a relationship with his son that is intimate and non-sexual. He should share his wisdom, encouragement, fears, triumphs and affirmation so that he may know and be known by his son. There is a need for male-male intimacy that is present in all men; we long to stand alongside each other and be found worthy. How else may we be judged worthy if we do not allow ourselves to be known?

Unfortunately, for those who have confused intimacy with sex, any expression of intimacy between men is interpreted as sexual. Many men were never taught how to be intimate with our male friends by our fathers or other male role models. Our culture has certainly done its best to create a view of masculinity that does not need intimacy, and Christian masculinity must reclaim intimacy as a human need. This maturing intimacy moves us toward sanctification.

In the absence of maturing intimacy, however, a man can move away from knowing and being known in such a way that he becomes less like Christ. This can be understood as *false intimacy*. False intimacy is a self-created illusion to avoid fear and pain resulting from a non-maturing intimacy. It is a desire for the other to be something they are not, or wanting more because of a sense that something is missing. Some might argue that the use of drugs or alcohol are ways that we can bypass the normal functioning of the body and attempt to get to a place of transcendence through chemical shortcuts.

Intimacy, however, is not to be sought indiscriminately. The cultivation of intimacy with several million people is a practical impossibility. Fortunately we are not called to seek to be intimate with every human being we come into contact with. We will have varying levels of intimacy with others. This is modeled in the life of Christ. We see a man that had several close friends, and he was exceptionally close to three in particular. While he did not have a wife, he was close with many women who knew him well. The intimate relationship that Jesus shared with his disciples as teacher and encourager was not a one-way street. He relied on his disciples in his ministry (Lk 9:1-2, Acts 1:8). There are many forms of intimacy and many appropriate, healthy ways to meet this need.

As Christians we believe that sexual intimacy between a husband and wife is characterized by passion, respect, trust and a selfless desire for the good of each other. But I believe we should avoid placing too much of an emphasis on sexual intercourse. To elevate it to a carnal "holy of holies" would be to deceive ourselves, only to find it hollow in its promise. Having a biblically sanctioned outlet for sexual intercourse and the regular practice of it in marriage is no guarantee that spiritual maturity will follow or that sanctification is assured. Neither is sexual intercourse the reward for marriage and able to solve all of a couple's problems. It is a means by which a husband and wife can share the journey of sanctification together, and it is also the means by which God can give the blessing of children according to his will. As a husband and wife share their bodies with one another they can experience the exclusivity of God's love and transcendence as they are in sexual union together.

I will be at the front of the line to confess that I believe that the marital covenant between a man and a woman can be a powerful force in the lives of a husband and wife, their children and those around them. But we should also remember that our value and identity does not come to us as a function of who we marry. Our value and identity is found in the image of God that we all bear and in Christ Jesus. Our journey can certainly be enhanced by marriage, but marriage and sexual fulfillment does not give us more worth nor is it a requirement for sanctification.

While it is important to not overemphasize the importance of sexual intimacy, it is also imperative that we not minimize it. It is not one of many biological functions that we should recklessly indulge in. It is not the scratching of a carnal itch that everyone is entitled to, nor should it be considered as necessary as eating or drinking. Sexual intimacy is not like every other biological function. It has significant consequences at every level of our existence: neurological, psychological, social and spiritual. And given that each one of us is a bio-psycho-socio-spiritual entity, it is no surprise that our sexual nature and how we express that nature has such wide-reaching implications.

LIVING SINGLE

Two issues regularly come up in my discussion of male sexuality with other men. The first is that many of these men are unmarried. When we are single, God calls us to live in sexual purity. In all of Scripture the only place where sexual relationships are sanctioned is within the marriage relationship between a man and a woman. This puts the single person in an awkward position. In order to engage in sexual activity Scripture reveals that two people must be in a marriage relationship. Unfortunately for many, this is not always the case. In our culture the average person gets married in their twenties (long after sexual maturation of the body), yet it is in the crucible of puberty when our sexual desires begin to surface as we discover the opposite sex.

Single men may understand their sexual longings as matters of intimacy, but they are anxious about the intensity of these sexual drives and wonder what options they have. An insensitive (but biblical) re-

sponse might be, "Get married." Paul admonishes the church at
Corinth to do so if they are unable to control these sexual drives
(1 Cor 7:9). In today's culture, however, this may be easier said than
done. Our culture promotes a view of marriage that is very different
from what Paul knew in the first century.

Having biblically sanctioned sex should not be the sole reason for
marrying. But does our culture foist a wrong understanding of marriage on men? Men are told to wait until they get their life in order,
find the most beautiful woman they can (special attention should be
paid to making sure her body maximally arouses him, that they
have "chemistry"), then somehow woo her to marry him. It is also
advisable to have a prenuptial agreement (to protect his assets given
the fifty percent chance of divorce). This view gives too great a
weight to "chemistry" and misses the importance of shared values
and commitments. The understanding of sex within marriage as imaging the exclusive love of God for his people is an example of this.
Many marriages built on emotional chemistry that ignore the importance of shared values do not last. After the flames of passion
fade, they are left with a mate that doesn't want what they want or
value what they value.

For those who chose mates based on shared values and commitments, the chemistry is more than just a flare which quickly goes
out. It is a spark which is fanned into a lifelong flame. Men should
not look for the first woman to marry them so that they can find a
release for their erotic energy. They may however need to reconsider
their understanding of what makes a godly marriage and reevaluate
how they look for a wife and any criteria they may have for a
spouse.

Within the context of married couples, Scripture speaks clearly to
what a healthy sexual relationship looks like. The duties of the man as
outlined in Ephesians 5:25-28 are quite clear: intentionality, honesty,
attention and time, giving of one's self and resources. There is mutual
consent and a controlled desire to be with the other. In addition to the
sharing of the body, there is sharing of emotions and an affirmation of

the other's worth. This kind of healthy sexuality does not destroy or corrupt either of the partners. It builds up each other, provides a sense of emotional and spiritual stability. It binds the two together. It is the antithesis of isolation; it is a form of communion.

The challenge for the single man is to find ways to continue on toward sanctification and ways to meet his needs for intimacy and sexual expression that do not dishonor himself, others or God's commands. This is best done in community through gleaning wisdom from other men, with mentors such as widowers and older single men.

MASTURBATION

A second issue that often haunts both single and married men is masturbation. You may be asking the question "Is all masturbation a sin?" I suggest that this is the wrong question to ask. It frames the question in such a way that we are trying to find out where the boundary lines are on a basketball court. It falls into the same category as "How far is too far when you are dating?"

The better question to ask is "Does masturbation lead me toward sanctification?' Masturbation (self-manipulation of the genitals to orgasm) is a common part of many men's sexual history. Some stumble into it as they discover their bodies, some are guided into it as they hear about it from their peers, and others have heard it preached against as though it is Satan's greatest tool against humanity. Men who compulsively masturbate (more than 2-3 times a week) can suffer from depression, memory problems, lack of focus, concentration problems, fatigue, back pain, decreased erections, premature ejaculation, and pelvic or testicular pain (Cooper et al., 2004, pp. 129-43; Carnes, 2001, pp. 45-78). Of all the forms of sexual acting out for men, masturbation is inherently the most isolating and potentially shaming.

Masturbation can take many forms. Men can become habitual (those who include it as part of their daily routine), compulsive (those who become preoccupied with it) or impulsive (those who feel a sudden urge to masturbate and cannot refrain) masturbators. In some cases, masturbation can be a symptom of a deeper problem—a problem not rooted in sin, but in our God-given need for intimacy. It can develop into a habit which, if repeated often enough, can become a compulsion which disrupts a man's ability to foster meaningful relationships. These relationships need not just be sexual with members of the opposite sex. It is not uncommon for men who compulsively masturbate to feel as if they are "less of a man." This feeling contributes to their sense that they would be seen as unworthy if their patterns of masturbation became known to their fellow men.

At the core of masturbation is that the self engages itself as an "other." The sexual act is intended as part of a relationship. Essentially, when a man masturbates he engages himself (or a better way of thinking of it is that he engages his body) in the sexual act. Masturbation, or self-stimulation, is different from manual stimulation by another person. When he is engaged in a sexual encounter with another person, it is truly a relationship (whether God-sanctioned or not). When a man stimulates himself, he treats himself as if he is two parts, mind and body. It is a fragmenting, disintegrating act. The mind is what experiences the ecstasy, the pleasure and the transcendence of the orgasm, and the body is the mechanism through which we bring ourselves to that place. The body is treated as a tool for the mind and neither respected nor honored as having its own intrinsic value.

This view of the self is a neo-Gnostic view. The reality of our oneness, our entire being as a singularity, is denied in the face of our desire to separate the mind from the body, the soul from the flesh. In this view the body is less important than the soul, and its desires are base and polluting. The body and its sexuality are partitioned and fractured which leads to psychological and spiritual distress.

THREE VIEWS OF MASTURBATION

In his book *The Struggle*, psychologist Steve Gerali offers three perspectives on masturbation. He suggests that each person should form their own view about masturbation based on the evidence of Scripture and scientific data (Gerali, 2003). The three positions are as follows.

1. *Masturbation is always* **sinful**. This position is the one that many Christians hold publicly. There are roundabout appeals to Scripture (it is not directly addressed) and church tradition to bolster this position. All instances of masturbation involve lust of the heart and/or mind that are inherently sinful. Masturbation occurs when a man fails to rely on God's chosen limits (intercourse with a spouse) to satisfy his sexual needs and longings.

2. *Masturbation is an issue of personal* **liberty** *(within responsible boundaries)*. There are passages which are used to make masturbation a wisdom issue. Romans 14:22-23 is used as a parallel between personal convictions about dietary restrictions and masturbation. This position holds that a man may determine if it is a sin issue for him, but he may not hold others to that standard, recognizing that others may or may not see it as a sin issue. The freedom that you have should not be flaunted lest it lead others who see it as sinful to stumble (Rom 14:13). There is a blanket of freedom to masturbate which reduces shame in the act (and also makes it less likely to be compulsive).

3. *Each instance requires* **discernment**. Masturbation is more of a situational ethic. There are times when it is sinful, and there are times when it is not. In the practice of discernment a man can know if he is free to masturbate or if to do so would be sinful. At times the lustful desires of the heart may make it sinful, but at other times it is the means by which God delivers them from sexual temptation—it can be God's gift. This position offers neither a blanket restriction nor a blanket freedom; discernment is exercised.

No matter which of these someone adheres to, each option leaves open the potential for masturbation to be sinful. In option #1 it is always a sin. In #2 as a matter of personal liberty, it is sinful if one goes outside the boundaries given by God and causes others to stumble. In #3 as a matter of discernment, it is sinful to knowingly masturbate when one believes it to be sinful and does anyway.

Some men believe that there is no physiological outlet other than releasing sperm (ejaculation, orgasm) as essential for relief. According to this logic, women must feel a release from these needs for sexual intimacy when they go through their menstrual cycle, and this is not always the case. But many men forget that God does provide a means of sexual release—the nocturnal emission. Unfortunately many men would rather masturbate than wait for this to occur. Because this occurs during sleep, there is limited chance of a behavioral problem occurring as a result of the emotional bonding to someone or something. In conversations with single men, I have heard reports that nocturnal emissions act as victories in the battle against compulsive masturbation. They recognize that God does provide for them and had failed to see his provision in this way.

Regardless of one's view on the moral dimension of masturbation, it has clear neurological consequences (Holstege, 2005, pp. 109-14; Holstege and Georgiadis, 2004, pp. 39-45; Holstege et al., 2003, pp. 9185-93). Masturbation is playing with neurochemical fire. It affects one emotionally and neurologically. For those who choose to view it as a matter of personal liberty or discernment, know that these effects will still be powerful. They may not have the same impact with respect to the shame that is felt afterwards (for those who view masturbation as a moral failure it has a greater risk of fueling an addictive or compulsive cycle), but it is not without consequences. You will be bound to something, because that is what it does neurologically—it associates the orgasm with something. The question to be asked is "*What* is it binding you to?"

There is a common misconception that masturbating doesn't affect a spouse (or future spouse), that there is a switch they can turn on or off without any consequences. This is simply not the case. One man reported to me that he was unable to climax with his wife after they were married because of his premarital masturbating. Unless she played out the scenarios that he had trained his mind to respond to (often including viewing pornography), he could not become sufficiently aroused to orgasm.

Another man shared with me that he would masturbate prior to sexual relations with his wife because it helped him delay orgasm when he was with his wife. "It's for her benefit I do it," he told me. "I can last longer. I can perform better."

"I wonder what she would say if you told her that," I responded. "Do you think she would be happy and thankful that you masturbate or do you think she would feel robbed?"

"Robbed. Robbed of what?"

"Robbed of the knowledge that she is the only one who sexually satisfies you and that you are connecting with her when you make love to her, not putting on a performance."

Because of the complexity of human sexuality we're able to develop associations between things that normally would not produce a sexual response and those things that do. For example, in my class I tell students that it would be easy to take any man and get him to a place where he could become sexually aroused by an item such as a baseball cap. Most students giggle at the thought of this, but it is actually quite easy to do. Imagine that I were to take a young man and have him watch sexually explicit videos on his computer for an hour a day across one month (I wouldn't actually do this, but some researchers have). Now imagine that I had placed a baseball cap on top of his computer monitor and asked him to leave it there during the month that we were doing the study. After a month's worth of watching the videos, if I presented my subjects with the same baseball cap, I would see a physiological response of sexual arousal (i.e., hormone release, increased heart rate, erection, etc.).

If we take this further, we can see how sexual fantasies or mentally replaying a satisfying sexual encounter can cause us to strengthen the connection between the particular object and our sexual arousal. If taken to its extreme, it leads to the development of fetishes. It is important to note, however, that for a person to have a fetish, sexual satisfaction occurs only with the object—the object becomes necessary for fulfillment as opposed to the baseball cap which has become a trigger for arousal.

For the single man, masturbating is how he trains himself in self-sufficiency with respect to his sexual needs. This is carried into marriage. For the married man, it betrays his commitment to allow his wife to meet his needs for intimacy. Unhealthy sexuality involves deception, selfishness and manipulation of individuals and circumstances. Unhealthy sexuality also robs you of the benefits of an intimate marriage. Although it feels as if it is a biological urge that is beyond control, our sexuality can and must be harnessed and directed. Self-control is mandated in Scripture and is necessary in order for us to have healthy, whole and fulfilling lives.

How do we bring God into the place which masturbation promises to fill yet does not satisfy? When we do, how quickly is God replaced by shame and guilt? There cannot be any disconnect from the body. If we try to disconnect ourselves from our bodies, regardless of our motives, it results in a fracturing of the person. Is there a time when masturbation becomes a form of self-rape? Not always. There are times when we knowingly and whole-heartedly engage in the behavior. But many men have reported that there are times when they are unable to stop themselves, pressured by an internal force that drives them toward doing something that they do not want to do. This leads them to believe there is something unfixable about them and leads them to a place of shame. This shame becomes a barrier to intimacy and a telling feature in the lives of many men who are caught in the machinery of pornography (Kwee, Dominguez and Ferrell, 2007).

DEFUSING SHAME

Individual instances of sinfulness are more easily dealt with, but addictive, compulsive, impulsive, selfish patterns are barriers to sanctification. All of us are sinful and have fallen short of the kingdom of God (Rom 3:23). No one gets it right all of the time. Holiness is not a place that you get to and then remain in permanently. My hope is that each man would embrace the sacredness of his sexuality. Regardless of each man's place in life, whether married or single, widowed or dating, the story of the gospel is about redemption. Allow that story to play itself out in your life in this area. With each failure, we confess and repent, then receive God's mercy and grace. Do not let shame imprison you—you are a child of the Most High. Our sexuality is a means through which we can taste the ecstasy that is found when we enter into communion with the transcendent Creator.

Regardless of our sexual history, we must always remember that there is no sin that the blood of Jesus Christ is unable to cleanse. The sacrifice of Christ may not restore physical consequences of our sin (or the sins that others commit against us), but we can still be counted as righteous. Many have failed sexually, but this failure is never final and does not hold ultimate power over us. That being said, many experience particular shame because of the nature of sexual sin. Only in the power of the Holy Spirit can we find freedom from shame. The solution is found in the knowledge of Jesus Christ as Lord and Savior who gives us victory over sin.

Because we are created by God with a sexual nature, our sexuality is a good thing. Far too often we consider sex as dirty, something that we should not talk about. In truth, our sexual nature gives us an incredible insight into the relational aspect of God. While our sexuality has an obvious design for having children, it is even more important for the establishment of a special bond of intimacy between a husband and wife. The call that God places on each of us as his children is a call to holiness. God calls us to a standard of purity and holiness that he requires. This standard is in our best interest.

We are built for intimacy, wired to know and to be known. We are also given the power of his Spirit to carry us through the storms of life. We are given the blood of Christ to cleanse and restore us from our sin.

REFERENCES

Ågmo, Anders. 2008. On the concept of sexual arousal: A simpler alternative. *Hormones and Behavior* 53, no. 2 (2): 312-14.

Ariely, D., and G. Loewenstein. 2006. The heat of the moment: the effect of sexual arousal on sexual decision making. *Journal of Behavioral Decision Making* 19, no. 2: 87.

Balswick, J. K., and J. O. Balswick. 1999. *Authentic human sexuality: An integrated Christian approach.* Downers Grove, IL: InterVarsity Press.

Carnes, Patrick J. 2001. Cybersex, courtship, and escalating arousal: Factors in addictive sexual desire. *Sexual Addiction & Compulsivity* 8, no. 1: 45-78.

Cooper, Al, David L. Delmonico, Eric Griffin-Shelley and Robin M. Mathy. 2004. Online sexual activity: An examination of potentially problematic behaviors. *Sexual Addiction & Compulsivity* 11, no. 3: 129-43.

Gerali, Steve. 2003. *The struggle.* Colorado Springs, CO: NavPress Publishing Group.

Holstege, G. 2005. Central nervous system control of ejaculation. *World Journal of Urololgy* 23, no. 2 (Jun): 109-14.

Holstege, G., and J. R. Georgiadis. 2004. The emotional brain: neural correlates of cat sexual behavior and human male ejaculation. *Progress in Brain Research* 143: 39-45.

Holstege, G., J. R. Georgiadis, A. M. Paans, L. C. Meiners, F. H. van der Graaf and A. A. Reinders. 2003. Brain activation during human male ejaculation. *Journal of Neuroscience* 23, no. 27 (Oct 8): 9185-93.

Kwee, Alex W., Amy W. Dominguez and Donald Ferrell. 2007. Sexual addiction and Christian college men: Conceptual, assessment, and treatment challenges. *Journal of Psychology and Christianity* 26 (1): 3-13.

McMinn, Lisa G. 2004. *Sexuality and holy longing: Embracing intimacy in a broken world.* San Francisco: Jossey-Bass.

Schaumburg, H. 1992. *False intimacy: Understanding the struggle of sexual addiction.* Colorado Springs, CO: NavPress.

White, R. E. O. 2001. Sanctification. In Walter Elwell, ed., *Evangelical dictionary of theology,* 2nd ed. Grand Rapids, MI: Baker Book House.

8

Rewiring and Sanctification

WE ARE EMBODIED AND EMBEDDED at a number of levels—physical, psychological, social and spiritual. We are made as God's agents in this world for his pleasure and for our own. We are made for each other, to be present and relational with one another. When we better understand who we are as human beings made in the image of God, we see better our created nature. We are made to be conformed to the image of Christ, to be sanctified. That process begins in this life. The decisions we make now affect the ongoing process of neural rewiring, our emotional state, our behavior, our embodied soul. As we think on the things that are good, noble and right we are *becoming* something: sanctified, conformed to the image of Christ.

Knowledge about our biological nature is not an excuse for sin. "My brain made me do it" or "Porn has messed up my brain so I can't help myself" are not get-out-of-jail-free cards. We are still responsible for our actions. As a man cultivates patterns of depravity, he diminishes his ability to bear God's image rightly. The knowledge that we get from Scripture and science should not be used to deny, justify, rationalize, minimize, normalize or celebrate the exercising of brokenness. It should be used to show compassion for those who have been propelled by the needs and design of their created nature down the path of depravity.

Rather than blame the needs, we should look at the process by which these needs drove us to depravity. These very same needs, however, can be reclaimed and redirected to travel the path of sanctification and holiness. Rather than resign ourselves to view our sexual nature as an impediment in the journey toward holiness, our sexuality should be reframed as a principal driving force toward sanctification. Rather than denigrate the neurobiological rooting of our psychological experience, we should use this knowledge about how we neurologically form emotional attachments as a necessary part of the process of sanctification.

How does a man become "addicted to holiness"? How does he cultivate his embodied nature to embrace sanctification? Many of the principles that govern all of spiritual formation have their impact in the brain. We can reframe recovery from pornography, sex addictions and compulsions as a process of rewiring, redemption and sanctification.

Many practical details about recovery from pornography addiction and sexual compulsion can be found elsewhere in books written by clinical psychologists, recovering addicts and counseling experts (see Appendix A for a list of online resources). In lieu of reinventing the recovery wheel, I defer to the texts I have cited in this book and the resources in Appendixes A and B as starting points for practical matters of recovery. What is critical, however, is understanding that the recovery of thought is rooted in the embodied brain and designed for the process of sanctification. As a result, it is a matter of spiritual formation.

RECOVERY AS SPIRITUAL FORMATION

We must open our eyes to see how God has been at work in us. Once we understand how we are made, we must support each other in a spirit of compassion and forgiveness. Every man who struggles with pornography needs wisdom from other men (and women) who can provide insight, comfort, strength and encouragement. The need will be great, especially at the beginning of the recovery and redemption processes. Neurological troughs of depravity are rarely changed overnight, since they were not formed overnight. The burden will be heavy, but we must serve the man who is repentant because he bears the image of God. By listening, offering insight into root problems, correcting false thoughts and lies, reminding them of their created nature and helping to illumine the true nature of God's love for us all, we provide the support that is needed to change course.

We are meant to live in a worthy way, and that way is not traveled alone. Men must be called to account regularly and rebuked in love when necessary. Correction is not to be feared but sought out by the man who longs to become holy and good. The challenge of accountability must always be rooted in a spirit of grace and focused on behavior. To condemn someone who is in the midst of a shame cycle only makes matters worse. If they are unable to hear that they have value as a child of God, they cannot progress toward recovery. The emphasis should be on changing the behavior.

We should help each other to envision the unique way that each of us will be conformed to the image of Christ. As we help each other prepare for the realities of our day, we must also have dreams about how God will use our unique experience, gifts and passions within the body of Christ to manifest his love in this world. Without being overly idealistic, dreams for marriage, work, family and ministry should be encouraged and empowered. By recognizing that each person will have their own unique journey and place in the body of Christ, we honor them. We can move beyond trying to fit any preconceived notions of what they "should have been" if they had only avoided their sin, and recognize that God can still demonstrate his love for them in a unique way. This path of confession, enlightenment, encouragement, challenge and vision respects the process of spiritual formation in the life of a man imprisoned by pornography, as well as everyone else.

CONFESSION

The first step that a man can take to free himself from the prison of pornography (or any other sexual sin) is to confess. Confession moves beyond denial, minimization, normalization, justification and rationalization to a right understanding of one's own brokenness. It refuses to celebrate and revel in the sin, and is the first step toward reestablishing communion with God and others. Because pornography has such an isolating effect on men who are intent on hiding their problem, it is important that this confession be more than between him and God. By confessing to another person, the isolating effect that porn has on a man will be reduced. When sin is shared with another person, a man is forced to expose his brokenness. How a man exposes this brokenness, however, is critical in the healing process. Only with a repentant heart that is completely broken can a man begin the process of true recovery.

Many men confess if they are caught, but they may not be repentant. They may feel guilty, but they may not be truly repentant. The measure by which a man can recover from a pornography problem is equal to his willingness to do the things that evidence repentance. If he tries to minimize, normalize, justify or rationalize, true healing will be slow and unlikely. He must be completely broken, as King David was when confronted by the prophet Nathan (2 Sam 12), in order to be restored. The consequences may not disappear, but he must be prepared to live with them and do what is necessary to make amends. It is essential that a man come to a true place of brokenness on this path. If he does not acknowledge his need for God, it is difficult for him to make any lasting progress in his recovery.

Confession is difficult for many men because it is an admission of failure. This is at odds with their understanding of their masculinity. Men don't fail and don't admit it if they do; to do so is a sign of weakness. As a result, it is important to confess to someone who is able to be a part of the healing process. Many men, when confronted with their pornography problem will confess it to their spouse or girlfriend. They do so because they are often the person with whom they have their deepest intimate connection. They reach out to the one whom they love the most for help. The consequences, however, can be disastrous.

Choosing whom to disclose your problem with pornography is a delicate process. The individual should be mature, supportive, wise, trustworthy, discrete, compassionate and emotionally resilient.

Many men will share with a relative, teacher, respected church leader, pastor or good friend. Regardless of who you choose, remember that the need for another human being to hear your sin and speak the forgiveness of Christ to you is part of being human and becoming sanctified.

ENLIGHTENMENT

Once you have confessed and have decided to follow the path of repentance, the next step is to assess what is at the root of the problem. This entails finding the reasons that you act out. It is an educational process whereby a man can be enlightened of his condition. This is best done as a historical analysis of his sexual and relational history (an example of a sexual survey/history is provided online at the book's website; see appendix B). By reviewing patterns of pornography use and seeing how his personality fits into the problem, he is better able to see how his sin has affected him and how his behaviors, thoughts and personality contribute to his problem. Also, wrong thinking can be corrected by rethinking the *imago Dei,* by acknowledging that he is embodied, and by realizing that his sexuality is for imaging God's exclusive love. Wrong thinking is often at the core of many men's problems and creates unnecessary stress, anxiety and shame. By rethinking his masculinity, sexuality and need for intimacy, he is better able to make sense of his condition.

Another important aspect of this enlightenment is to identify the environmental, emotional, psychological and autonomic triggers that drive the sexual addiction, compulsion or impulse problem. This is best done with a mentor or counselor—someone who is able to provide wise insight from a relatively objective standpoint.

One thing that I do with many of the men I work with is use the principle of chaining. Chaining is a process that helps men identify their triggers. It helps them examine how their responses occur in a sequence. When someone I am mentoring acts out, I ask them to journal their day in a backwards fashion so that we can look for patterns of maladaptive behavior or distorted thinking. This journaling forces men to stop and seize the moment. Too many men go through their day at full speed and do not engage in disciplines of contemplation and self-reflection. When a man is forced to slow down and put his thoughts and feelings to paper, he learns the skill of reflection. This reflection enables him to better name his emotions, understand his motives, and act on what he has learned about himself.

Consider the following example of Tom. Tom is a single man in his twenties who had significant problems with pornography and masturbation. After viewing pornography and sexually acting out he wrote in his journal and reviewed the previous twenty-four hours.

1. Last night I was up late working on a project for work. I went to bed around 3 a.m.

2. I got up on time for work, but was tired.

3. My project was not well received by my boss at our 9 a.m. meeting.

4. I avoided my boss the rest of the morning. Avoiding him put me on edge.

5. The new woman in accounting smiled at me when she dropped off a report.

6. I found myself fantasizing about her, and I got an erection.

7. I wanted to see her again, so I made up a reason to stop off at her office and started flirting with her.

8. My boss walked by while I was flirting and ripped into me about the project again.

9. I was embarrassed and knew she would never be attracted to me or want to have sex with me.

10. I went back to my desk and fumed about my boss. I wanted to quit or find a way to get back at him.

11. Everyone left the office for a working lunch, but I made up an ex-

cuse to stay behind. I closed the blinds on my windows and locked the office door. I thought viewing porn would be a good way to get back at my boss.

12. Viewing the pictures gave me an erection, and I really felt the need to masturbate.

13. I viewed the pictures until someone knocked on the door. The images on the screen seemed to take forever to disappear.

14. It was my boss. He asked why the door was locked and was suspicious of what I was doing. I told him I was working on revisions to the report. He told me the next report had better be up to his standards.

15. I realized I was perspiring excessively and thought I smelled of sex. I felt like I had narrowly avoided being caught and erased the files from my computer.

16. I was preoccupied with my body odor for the rest of the afternoon.

17. The new woman from accounting brought the new report back right before 5 p.m. I reeked of sweat and was sure she could smell it.

18. I fantasized about her the entire drive home and had an erection.

19. My roommate wasn't home and had left a note saying he would be gone for the weekend.

20. While changing from my work clothes I was reminded of my body odor, the smell of sex, again.

21. I undressed, closed the blinds to the windows, locked the apartment, got some tissue paper, then went online. I knew I was going to view porn and I didn't care.

22. I surfed for hardcore images of secretaries for about 10 minutes (I knew right where to go because I've been there before). I found a video clip of a secretary that looked like the new accountant.

23. I looped the video for a couple of minutes, masturbating to it.

24. I smelled even more of sweat when I was done, so I took a shower.

25. I felt miserable and trapped. I was disgusted with myself.

A review of this chain yields a number of clear trigger points in Tom's day and the night before which contributed to his problem. The stress from his job, lack of sleep, ritualized pattern of acting out (undressing, closing the blinds, locking the door), body awareness (the smell of his sweat tied to his acting out) and sexual preoccupation/ interest in his coworker (his surfing for secretary clips) were clear to me, but not to him.

Tom did not see how they were related to each other, how these small drips throughout his day had become a current of sexual compulsion coursing through the neural troughs of his brain. This process of journaling and backtracking the chain of events is helpful to identify the issues and begin to formulate a plan to aid in recovery. When a man is enlightened to his stumbling blocks, he is able to intentionally organize his life and his thoughts to avoid the neurological troughs of pornography and sexual acting out. He redirects these thoughts, channeling his sexual energy toward sanctification. By making some rather nominal changes in his day that had little to do with sex per se (not procrastinating on projects, getting enough sleep, staying at his desk, having lunch with friends, having a stick of deodorant in his office desk drawer, leaving the blinds at his apartment open), Tom was able to interrupt this maladaptive pattern.

By discovering their sexual triggers that initiate a compulsion or impulse, men can identify them before they progress to a point where they lose the ability to control their behavior. Short-circuiting the rituals breaks men out of their compulsive cycles and avoids situations that may make impulses more difficult to resist. Once a man finds out what triggers his patterns, he can organize his world to reduce the chances of returning to the old trough of porn and acting out.

CHALLENGE

The presence of an ongoing mentoring relationship with an older, wiser and more mature man has a significant impact on psychological well-being. A mentor is someone deliberately chosen whom you see as modeling a life that is on the path toward sanctification. A mentor serves not only as guide but as a model of one who has become conformed to the image of Christ. Finding someone who has traveled on the same paths that you have helps a man deal with the challenges he is facing and helps anticipate those yet to come. Only those who know a man well can tell when he is lying, and only those who care for him deeply will call him out when he is.

Often men look for accountability with their peers, but a man needs a mentor to give him wisdom that his peers cannot. Peers may struggle with the same issues, be unaware of their own flaws, overestimate their knowledge of the problem or not have enough life experience to make sense of it all. Men who surround themselves with their peers and proudly refuse to accept the counsel of their elders fall into a locker room mentality. In the locker room mentality, peers go through the motions of accountability; they all know they are lying, but no one wants to call another out lest he be called out. This accountability has no substance, no bite, and is the sign of a shallow relationship. Many of these peer accountability relationships eventually dissolve.

A mentor is someone who has dealt with the trials and challenges and found redemption. Just as a team needs a coach to keep them honest, so should a man have someone he respects and can learn from, walking with them along the path to holiness. When the relationship is deep and life-encompassing, our lives are spent in community. When the relationship is deep enough a mentor can tell when a man is stumbling. He can see that trouble is approaching and warn a man about an upcoming battle.

Men were created for relationships with women, and they were also created for relationships with each other. The myths of masculinity in our culture have isolated men from each other and impaired their ability to honor and bless one another. Too many men have too few intimate male friends. Their friendships run only as deep as the things they do together. By finding male friends to go deeper with, the need for intimacy can be met in nonsexual ways with these male friends. When this happens the intensity of the need for intimacy is not funneled through sexual intercourse with a woman; it can be shared across many relationships. Sexual intimacy may be experienced with one woman, but intimacy can be experienced with others as well. Not all intimacy is genital, so do not feel restricted in your relationships with your brothers in Christ.

In some cases it may become necessary to seek professional help with a severe problem with pornography. There are those whom God has gifted and trained to deal with severe problems and are equipped to handle the messiness of life. It is a calling that they have for those who have exercised their brokenness or who have experienced severe woundedness. There is no shame in seeking out a professional therapist or getting involved in treatment program that specializes in helping people break free from bondage to sexual sin. A psychological evaluation may reveal additional problems which have gone undetected. Not all mentors are trained in clinical psychology, and the need for someone with these skills may be necessary.

Another opportunity for healing is in the reestablishing of relationships that were lost. Pornography isolates, and men often neglect previously valued friendships. In the case of a spouse (or others) feelings of betrayal, distrust, abandonment and disillusionment will need to be repaired. A spouse may have been compared or compared herself to porn models, and her self-esteem may be battered. She may avoid intimacy with her husband or remain emotionally detached during sexual intimacy. If the user has blamed the partner for his problem or involved his wife in viewing pornography, significant emotional damage may have occurred. The wife may overcompensate emotionally and try to win back her husband by attempting to be more sexually available or to reduce the severity of the consequences. Or his wife may no longer want to have sex with him because of her anger and distrust. Fears of disease (if there has been adultery) or that the user is now at risk to sexual assault or molest of children must also be addressed.

As part of humanity's fallen nature, objectifying one another happens all too often. But the question is whether you want objectifying others to become a habit that is neurologically so hardwired that you cannot prevent yourself from doing it. The question is whether you want to train yourself in such a way that you become neurologically wired so that your reflex is to see every woman as a person and not an object.

When this happens, the drifting of your eyes to evaluate her ability to sexually arouse you or sizing her up as a sexual partner will be so out of place that it will be easily identified. Once identified, it can be captured and discarded. Once discarded, an internal celebration of taking another step along the path of sanctification is in order. As we take each thought captive to weigh its place in the journey toward sanctification or depravity, we become coworkers with the Holy Spirit in the making of the mind of Christ in ourselves.

Imagine that you could be neurologically "enslaved" to purity rather than porn. Enslaved to seeing the dignity of each individual rather than their utility to you. This is the distinction between the journey toward sanctification and the journey toward depravity. As you travel farther along either road, you pick up momentum and it becomes harder to turn around. The farther down the road you travel, the less opportunity you have to deviate from the road as it narrows. The road to depravity leads into the heart of hell and yields isolation. The road toward sanctification, however, leads into the heart of God and yields freedom from temptation.

Some of the best coaches and managers in professional sports are not just those who can come up with a good game plan, but are able to change their plan as the game is in progress. As you go through recovery and healing, don't be afraid to let go of things that are not beneficial to you. If you find that journaling is tedious and stressful and increases your shame, stop doing it. If you find that listening to classical music soothes your soul and relieves work-related tension, listen to it. Because you have a unique personal history, you will have a unique path to recovery as well. Do not expect that what works for someone else must work with you. Do not expect that what doesn't work for someone else won't work for you either.

ENVISIONING SANCTIFICATION

Some questions you may ask are, "How does recovery take place? Can my brain be retrained to respond appropriately? Is there any neuropsychological evidence for it?" These are the right questions to be asking. How does recovery take place? It takes place in community and is rooted in changing your embodied nature—most notably by rewiring the patterns of sexual arousal and response in the brain. Can someone retrain their brain to respond in an appropriate manner to sexual arousal? Most certainly, but this must be informed by the mandates of Scripture and the wisdom found in the body of Christ. This must be empowered by the Holy Spirit. This empowering, however, might be a little less mystical and more embodied than most of us think it is.

Is there any neuropsychological evidence that any of this is real? I hope that the scientific studies that I cited have had been at least somewhat convincing. There is little research being done on the neurological basis of porn addiction. In part this is because it is not seen as necessary. Pornography is legal and acknowledging it as harmful is not politically convenient, so there are not many federal grants to fund research on it; that is the social reality. My research group at Wheaton College has begun a number of studies to address these very questions. I am looking forward to sharing that research in the near future, so stay tuned if you want more data.

Much of this book has been focused on reevaluating our understanding of how we are made, how we are wired and what we are made for. What may start off as a seemingly innocent lingering on a nude image can lead to a mind consumed by pornography. An unhealthy pattern of depravity can develop if a man isn't careful. But the very thing that leads him down this path is the same thing that can lead him out of depravity and into holiness.

Every man and woman is an embodied creation who is intended to become sanctified in the image of Jesus Christ. As each man comes to understand who he is, how he is uniquely made and what he is intended for, he comes to know himself and his Creator more rightly. Each of his struggles becomes a part of the unique path that enables him to manifest God's love to others.

As a man uses his sexuality to propel him toward sanctification, it involves his embodied nature. The small decisions that he makes set the stage whereby he limits his abilities to entertain sin and temptation. This process is not just a spiritual one, but involves the way that his brain is neurologically wired. These small decisions—the impact of a sexual encounter with a wife—the proper seeing of women as made in the image of God, are stored neurologically as circuits that aid in our sanctification. By understanding our purpose in this life and by demonstrating and experiencing God's love, we are conformed to the image of Christ. We see the image of God in each person, we are able to appreciate women without consuming them, and we move beyond objectification to real relationship, presence and intimacy.

The process of sanctification is an addiction to holiness, a compulsive fixation on Christ and an impulsive pattern of compassion, virtue and love. This is what we are wired for. This is what we are meant for.

Appendix A

Resources for Recovery from
Online Pornography and Sex Addiction

Wired for Intimacy
http://wiredforintimacy.blogspot.com
Website for resources related to the *Wired for Intimacy* book. Updates on the most recent brain research related to pornography and recovery.

XXXchurch.com
www.xxxchurch.com
XXXchurch is designed to bring awareness, openness and accountability to those affected by pornography. XXXchurch.com exists to help those who are in over their heads with pornography, both consumers and those in the industry. Staff tour the world speaking at colleges, churches and community centers.

National Coalition for the Protection of Children & Families
www.nationalcoalition.org
An organization designed to move the people of God to embrace, live out, preserve and advance the truth of biblical sexuality.

New Life Partners
www.newlifepartners.org
A support group for wives whose husbands are caught in the web of sexual addiction.

Pure Life Ministries

www.purelifeministries.org

Pure Life Ministries helps men who are struggling with sexual addiction. Pure Life Ministries has been leading men into purity since 1986.

Be Broken Ministries

www.bebroken.com

A ministry designed to help men and women live every day in sexual purity and provide support and resources to help live a life of sexual purity.

LIFE (Living in Freedom Everyday) Ministries

www.freedomeveryday.org

Articles cover what sexual addiction is, why overcoming it is important, the difference between love and sex addiction, and assessment for self-diagnosis.

Pure Online

www.pureonline.com

An online sex and pornography addiction recovery resources site which utilizes online workshops.

Operation Integrity

www.operationintegrity.org

OI is a Christ-centered twelve-step fellowship that helps men and women recover from sex/porn addiction, helping them to become healthy, balanced and well-integrated with Jesus Christ and others.

Bethesda Workshops

www.bethesdaworkshops.org

A Christian-based ministry that offers clinical treatment for pornography and other forms of sexual addiction.

Appendix B

Books on Pornography and Sex Addiction Recovery

Arterburn, S., F. Stoeker and M. Yorkey. 2000. *Every man's battle: Winning the war on sexual temptation one victory at a time.* Colorado Springs, CO: Waterbrook Press.

Bowring, Lyndon, ed. 2005. *Searching for intimacy.* Waynesboro, GA: Authentic Media.

Carnes, P. 2001. *Out of the shadows: Understanding sexual addiction.* Center City, MN: Hazelden Publishing & Educational Services.

Carnes, P. 1991. *Don't call it love: Recovery from sexual addiction.* New York: Bantam Books.

Carnes, P. J., D. L. Delmonico and E. Griffin. 2007. *In the shadows of the net: Breaking free from compulsive online sexual behavior.* Center City, MN: Hazelden Publishing & Educational Services.

Cooper, Al. 2000. *Cybersex: The dark side of the force.* Philadelphia: Brunner-Routledge,.

Jensen, R., G. Dines, G. Dines, R. Jensen and A. Russo. 1998. *Pornography: The Production and Consumption of Inequality.* Philadelphia: Routledge.

Sbraga, T. P., and T. O. D. William. 2003. *The sex addiction workbook: Proven strategies to help you regain control of your life.* Oakland, CA: New Harbinger Publications.

Schaumburg, H. 1992. *False intimacy: Understanding the struggle of sexual addiction.* Colorado Springs, CO: Navpress.

Willingham, Russell. 1999. *Breaking free: Understanding sexual ad-*

diction & the healing power of Jesus. Downers Grove, IL: InterVarsity Press.

Young, K. S. 2001. *Tangled in the web: Understanding cybersex from fantasy to addiction.* Bloomingon, IN: Authorhouse.

Young, K. S. 1998. *Caught in the net: How to recognize the signs of internet addiction—and a winning strategy for recovery.* New York: Wiley.

Index